# Atlas of Manipulative Techniques for the Cranium & Face

# Atlas of Manipulative Techniques for the Cranium & Face

Alain Gehin
Illustrated by Dominique Linglin

Eastland Press
SEATTLE

Originally published as *Atlas des Techniques Manipulatives des Os du Crane et de la Face.* Copyright 1981, Maisonneuve.


English translation © 1985 by Eastland Press, Incorporated, P.O. Box 99749, Seattle, Washington 98139 www.info@eastlandpress.com
All rights reserved
Library of Congress Card Number: 85-80135
International Standard Book Number: 0-939616-02-5
Printed in the United States of America


Typography by Franklin & Welker, Incorporated, Chicago, Illinois.
Jacket design by Patricia O'Connor.

10  9

The author would like to express his special thanks to Dominique Linglin, who has taught anatomy in the European College of Etiopathy, for his artistic participation and most charming personality.

Without his talent, his broad knowledge and his insight, this work would not have been so instructive. His art, informed by his precise understanding of anatomy and articular physiology, has made the book more lively and cogent.

The author would also like to thank Anne-Marie Louise for her assistance in translating this work into English.

# Table of Contents

# Foreword

The most effective practitioner is one who understands anatomy and physiology, and has the tactile sensitivity to provide an acute awareness of the inherent forces operating in the patient under his or her hands. Such a practitioner can then devise the technique which will permit the inherent therapeutic potency to resolve the dysfunction.

The teaching of techniques applicable to the cranial mechanism must therefore be preceded by a profound study of the anatomy of the central nervous system, the reciprocal tension membrane (i.e., the dura mater with its folds, attachments and venous sinuses, and the fluctuant motility of the cerebrospinal fluid), as well as the intricate anatomical form of every cranial bone. It is M. Gehin's assumption that this book will be used by those already equipped with this knowledge of the primary respiratory mechanism. In cooperation with M. Linglin, he has provided a clear rendering of the position of the practitioner's hands on the head for the diagnosis and treatment of membranous articular strains of the cranial base. The forces and axes around which the bones move are clarified for the student by these excellent line drawings.

This volume describes many techniques, all of which may be of great value to certain patients in the hands of certain practitioners. But let it never be supposed that this is all-inclusive. To accomplish change, the practitioner must be ever alert to the needs of this patient at this moment and must respond creatively to them, designing the appropriate technique indicated by the relative size and build of patient and practitioner; by the forces traumatically imposed on that mechanism under his or her hands; and by the strength and vitality of the inherent therapeutic potency within.

Students of the cranial concept will find in this volume vivid visual reminders of hand positions for diagnosis of the various sphenobasilar strains, and for the treatment of peripheral articular dysfunctions.

We thank the author and the artist for this valuable contribution to the literature on the cranial concept.

In the final analysis remember that the "thinking, feeling, seeing, knowing fingers" that apply this teaching are the key to the patient's restoration to a state of well-being.

*May 1985*                           — *Viola M. Frymann, D.O., F.A.A.O.*
                                     *Chairperson, Department of Osteopathic Principles and Practice*
                                     *College of Osteopathic Medicine of the Pacific*

# Editors' Preface

This book is the product of a European manipulative perspective on various techniques for treating the cranium and the face. While, as M. Gehin writes in his Preface, many of these techniques are familiar to American and British practitioners who utilize the cranial concept, some of the techniques are either derived from other traditions or are performed in slightly different ways. Just as craniosacral practitioners ask their colleagues and patients to keep an open mind about the cranial concept, we ask the reader to be receptive to techniques that may seem at variance with standard conceptions of craniosacral therapy. There is room for variation in all therapeutic systems that attempt to deal with the complex nature of human health and disease. Every school and style offers its unique perspective.

A major portion of M. Gehin's contribution has been to gather together techniques from various traditions. Although we urged M. Gehin to identify the source of each technique, he declined, believing that such attribution was impertinent and could be misleading inasmuch as the techniques were best regarded as belonging to a common heritage.

The author's collaborator, M. Linglin, has illustrated the techniques collected in this book with skill and style. While the illustrations are self-explanatory, we have found it necessary to adapt the text to the needs of an English-speaking audience. In cooperation with M. Gehin, we have clarified and amplified some of the concepts in the French edition of this work, and made changes in the terminology to be more consistent with other English texts.

Nevertheless, we have preserved some of the differences that all of us believe are very important. One of the major differences in terminology between this book and most other cranial texts in English is that M. Gehin uses the words 'expansion' and 'relaxation' to describe the general motion of the cranial rhythm. The expansion phase of the cranial rhythm is equivalent to 'flexion' and the relaxation phase to 'extension'. M. Gehin confines the use of the terms flexion or extension, and external rotation or internal rotation to describing the motion of particular bones. His use of these terms emphasizes the physiologic motion of the cranial rhythm, and assists the student in understanding and remembering the essential nature of the cranial mechanism.

Another important difference is that M. Gehin, unlike many English-speaking practitioners, believes that it is easier (especially for novices) to achieve a release if the techniques are performed during the expansion (i.e., flexion) phase of the cranial rhythm, when most of the sutures have a tendency to expand.

Most of the techniques that M. Gehin presents in this book are based upon the cranial concept. Part of that concept is that the practitioner's goal is to potentiate the patient's own self-healing mechanisms. In order to do this the cranial mechanism must be approached gingerly and gently. Readers should therefore remember that, unless otherwise specifically noted, movements are always subtle and pressure always very slight.

Manipulative techniques cannot be learned solely from a book. As an atlas of techniques, this book assumes that the reader already has a sound foundation in anatomy, and some facility with manipulation in general and with craniosacral therapy in particular. We value the unique perspective of M. Gehin and the talents of M. Linglin. It is our hope that this English language edition of their book will be of interest and use to many practitioners.

*May 1985*                    *— Hugh A. O'Connor*
                              *Dan Bensky, D.O.*

                                   *Editors*

# Preface

This presentation of cranial manipulative techniques requires some preliminary remarks.

Cranial manipulative movement is induced by the practitioner's fingers. This movement, though amplified by the flexibility of the bones of the living organism (especially those of the vault) depends upon the shape of these bones and on the specific disposition of the articular surfaces. Moreover, the least complex bone of the cranium presents several joints which are often situated in different spatial planes. Movement is possible only if the manipulations take into account the almost simultaneous movement of all the other cranial joints. Even partial failure to do this can lead to errors that result in lesions.

The acquisition of these techniques requires a particularly precise and minute knowledge, the education for which in no circumstances should ever be abbreviated or circumvented. No manipulative training can be forged in haste, especially in this field where everything acts at a most subtle level. Mastering the right and reasoned gesture is achieved only through time and practice.

The manipulations described in this atlas have been chosen for their efficacy; they have been tested through extensive application in quite varied times and geographic areas. Although several of them have been described by British and American writers (including Sutherland, Magoun, Lippincott, Arbuckle, Lake, Cottam and De Jarnette), several others have been collected by the author in Europe as well as in Asia and Oceania. These are techniques taught at the European College of Etiopathy in Geneva, within the framework of that school's original philosophy of manual medicine.

This work does not pretend to be exhaustive, or anything other than a teaching tool. Except when otherwise stated, the descriptions are presented with a view to the direct correction of a lesion. The theory upon which these manipulations are based is not systematically discussed here. These relatively simple techniques should always be adapted to the particular patient at the moment of application.

In oriental philosophy there is a saying, "When the pupil is ready, the master appears." May this atlas prompt the pupil along his or her own path of discovery.

# Summary Illustrations

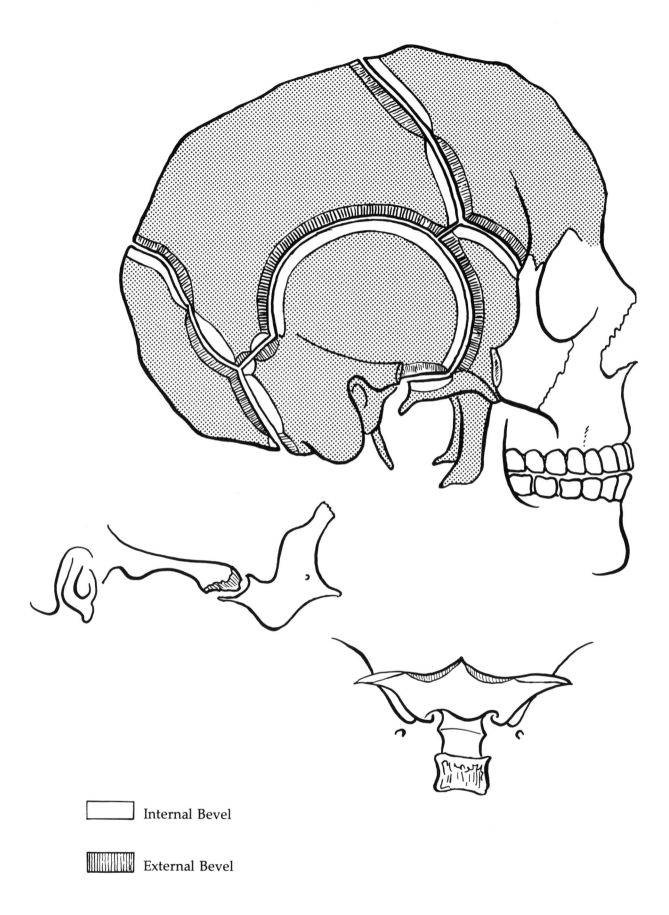

**Bevels of the Cranial Bones**

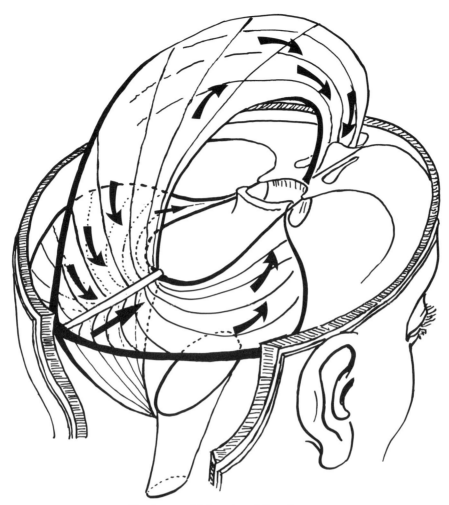

**Reciprocal Tension Membrane**

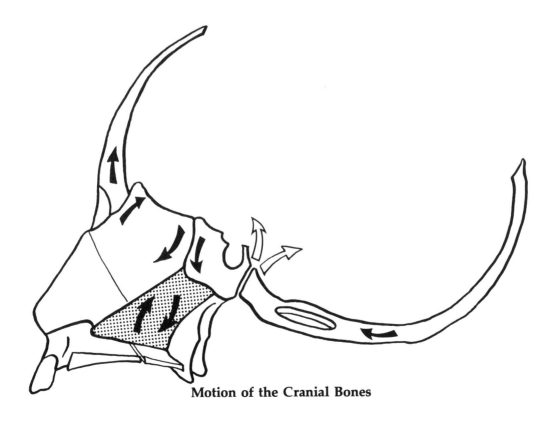

**Motion of the Cranial Bones**

# I General Techniques

This chapter includes all the techniques which have a direct and immediate effect on the general cranial motion, also called the cranial rhythmic impulse. These involve multiple contacts on each of the principal bones of the cranium. When the practitioner's fingers are completely passive, these techniques can also serve as part of a diagnostic examination.

We have combined these techniques with those involving manipulation of most of the sutures, as well as those having a general effect on the reciprocal tension membrane.

We have also included in this chapter the cranial manipulative techniques that affect the entire body.

The manipulative techniques which are described in this work provide only a framework of reference for the practitioner. As with all manual techniques, the therapeutic action must be adapted not only to the patient's biomechanics, but to the practitioner's as well. It is desirable that the reader not feel constrained to follow precisely the models described in this text, but use these models to develop a personal style within the wide range of possibilities and variations.

We begin this descriptive approach with the two principal vault holds for the cranium. Both of these allow for the use of a certain number of different general techniques, the choice of which in each case being specifically determined by the patient's situation, by convenience, or by the practitioner's skill.

# VAULT HOLD

## Objectives

- To assess the general motion of the bones of the cranium; to appraise the freedom of motion of the cranial base.
- To normalize motion in both the cranial base and vault.
- To assess the degree of participation (whether physiological or pathological) of each bone in the general motion of the cranium.

## Position of the patient

Supine, comfortable and relaxed.

The patient should remove glasses, any objects in pockets, and any nonfixed dental appliances.

## Position of the practitioner

Seated at the patient's head, forearms resting on the treatment table adjusted to a convenient height. The fingers of both hands are held without tension and spread out in space, forming a hollow in which the patient's cranium can be placed.

## Points of contact

The pads of the finger tips touch the patient's cranium, on each side, in the following manner:

- the little finger, almost parallel to the occipital curve, meets the squamous part of the occiput at the lateral angles;
- the ring finger, behind the ear at the asterion, is placed on the parietal posteroinferior angle (middle joint) and on the temporal mastoid region (distal joint);
- the middle finger, in front of the ear, touches with its middle joint (or distal, depending on the shape of the patient's cranium and on the size of the practitioner's hand) at the antero-inferior parietal angle (pterion); the fingertip is placed on the zygomatic process of the temporal bone;
- the index finger is placed on the greater wing of the sphenoid; (For certain techniques, the index finger is placed in a more anterior position, behind the external orbital process of the frontal. If the practitioner's hands are small relative to the size of the patient's head, the index fingers may contact the lateral angles of the frontal.)
- the thumbs rest against each other above the cranium, forming a base for the flexor muscles of the fingers.

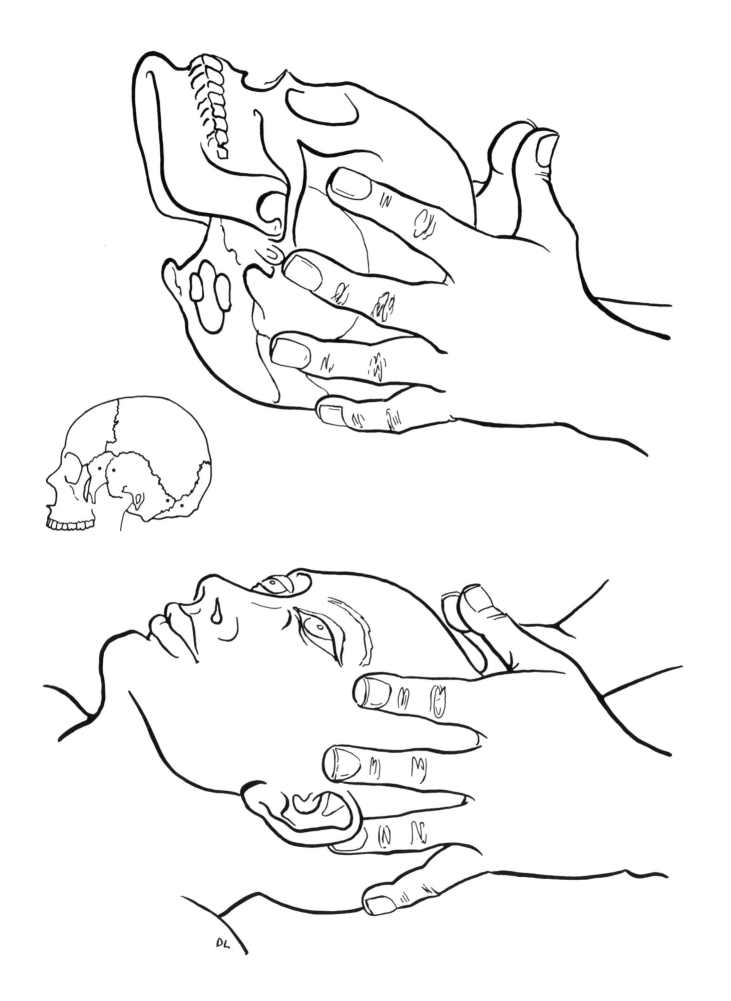

DL

# FRONTO-OCCIPITAL HOLD

### Objectives

The same as those described for the vault hold (page 10). The different contacts allow the practitioner to use whichever approach is therapeutically appropriate.

### Position of the patient

Supine, comfortable and relaxed.

The patient should remove glasses, any objects in pockets, and any nonfixed dental appliances.

### Position of the practitioner

Seated to the right or left of the patient's head, lower hand resting on the table top adjusted to a convenient height. This hand holds the patient's occipitosquama area. The upper hand is placed over the frontal bone.

### Points of contact

Lower hand: cupped so as to hold the patient's occiput with the tips of the fingers on the opposite occipital angle. The angle of the occipital squama closest to the practitioner rests on the thenar and/or hypothenar eminences.

Upper hand: also forming a cup, enveloping the frontal bone without touching it; making contact with the two external surfaces of the greater wings of the sphenoid. Thus:

— the pad of the tip of the index finger and/or middle finger is on the side opposite the practitioner; and

— the pad of the tip of the thumb is on the practitioner's side.

If the practitioner's hand is small relative to the patient's head, it may contact the lateral angles of the frontal bone.

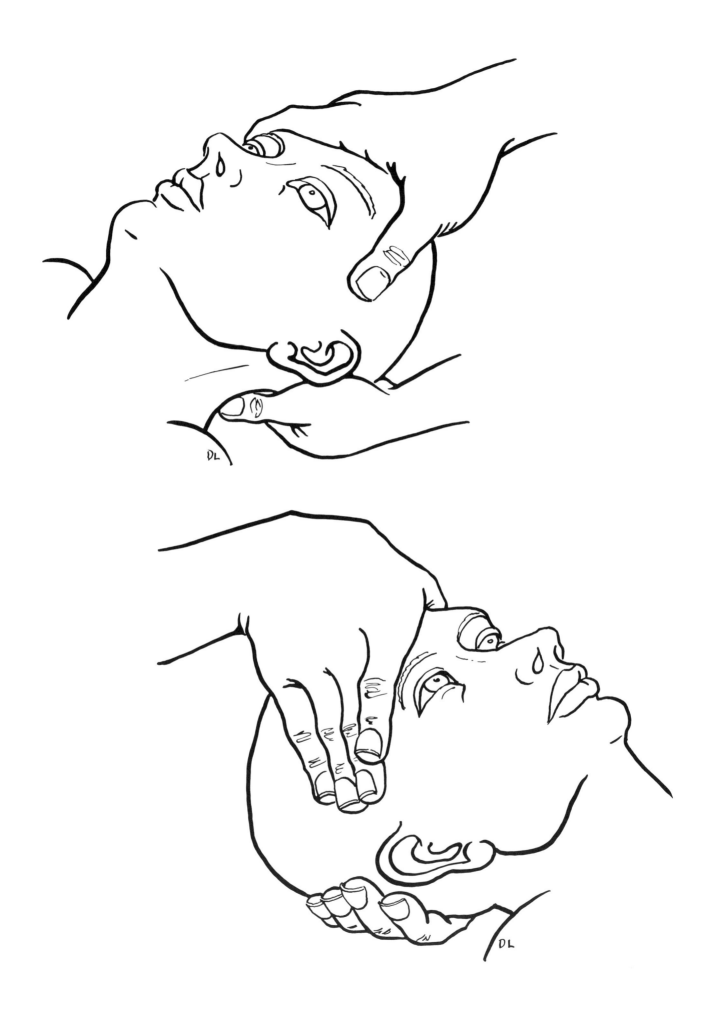

# FLEXION PHASE OF THE CRANIAL MOTION

## VAULT HOLD

### Objectives

- To assess the mobility of the cranial mechanism during flexion (and therefore during external rotation).
- To directly correct an extension lesion.
- To indirectly correct a flexion lesion.
- To assess the amount of motion of any particular cranial bone, within the context of the cranial motion as a whole, during the expansion phase of the cranial mechanism.

### Movement

Using the vault hold (page 10), the practitioner proceeds in the following manner. During the expansion phase of the cranial mechanism, those portions of the ring and middle fingers on the lateral angles of the occiput or the parietal angles are drawn caudally and laterally; while the index fingers, on the greater wings of the sphenoid, are shifted anteriorly and caudally.

### Comments

When contact on the greater wings of the sphenoid is uncomfortable or even painful for the patient (as in cases of temporal arteritis), it is sufficient to lay the index fingers behind the external orbital process of the frontal bone, to induce this bone to carry out a flexion movement (external rotation) during the expansion phase of the cranium.

It is important to remember that this is not an active movement on the part of the practitioner; it is a process of determining the inherent motion that is occurring within the mechanism. This applies as well to the extension phase which follows.

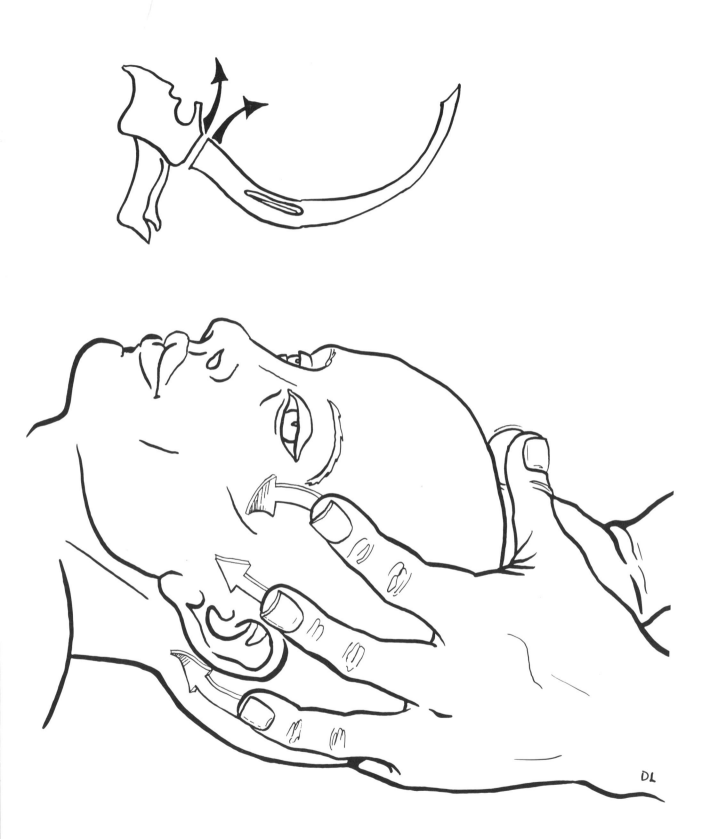

# FLEXION MOVEMENT

## FRONTO-OCCIPITAL HOLD

### Objectives

- To assess the amount of inherent cranial motion during flexion (and therefore during external rotation).
- To directly correct an extension lesion.
- To indirectly correct a flexion lesion.
- To assess the amount of motion of any particular cranial bone, within the context of the cranial motion as a whole, during the expansion phase of the cranial mechanism.

### Movement

Using the fronto-occipital hold (page 12), the practitioner proceeds in the following manner. During the expansion phase of the cranial mechanism, simultaneously:

- the lower hand, under the occiput, brings it caudally and anteriorly, in a circular movement around its transverse axis;
- the upper hand draws the greater wings of the sphenoid anteriorly and caudally, around its transverse axis.

### Comment

When the upper hand grips the greater wings of the sphenoid, the practitioner should avoid putting any pressure on the frontal bone which could induce a paradoxical movement.

When the upper hand has made its contact behind the external orbital process of the frontal bone, it should execute the same movement as described above around its transverse axis. However, the palm of the hand pressing on the frontal bone should press on the upper part of the metopic suture in order to more fully appreciate the motion.

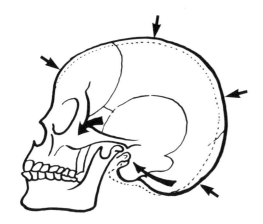

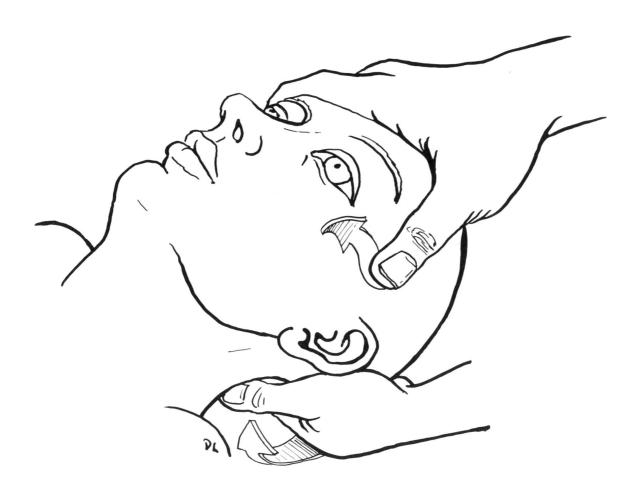

# EXTENSION MOVEMENT

## VAULT HOLD

### Objectives

- To assess the degree of inherent cranial motion during extension (and therefore during internal rotation).
- To directly correct a flexion lesion.
- To indirectly correct an extension lesion.
- To assess the freedom of motion of any particular cranial bone, within the context of the cranial motion as a whole, during the extension or relaxation phase of the cranial mechanism.

### Movement

Using the vault hold (page 10), the practitioner proceeds in the following manner. This movement is the opposite of the flexion movement. During the relaxation phase of cranial motion, the middle and little fingers on the parietals and occiput move cephalad and medially, while simultaneously the index fingers on the greater wings of the sphenoid move in a cephalad and posterior direction.

### Comment

If the practitioner has placed his index fingers behind the external orbital process of the frontal bone, he or she should execute a circular movement around the transverse axis, drawing the lateral angles of the frontal bone in a posterior, cephalad and medial direction.

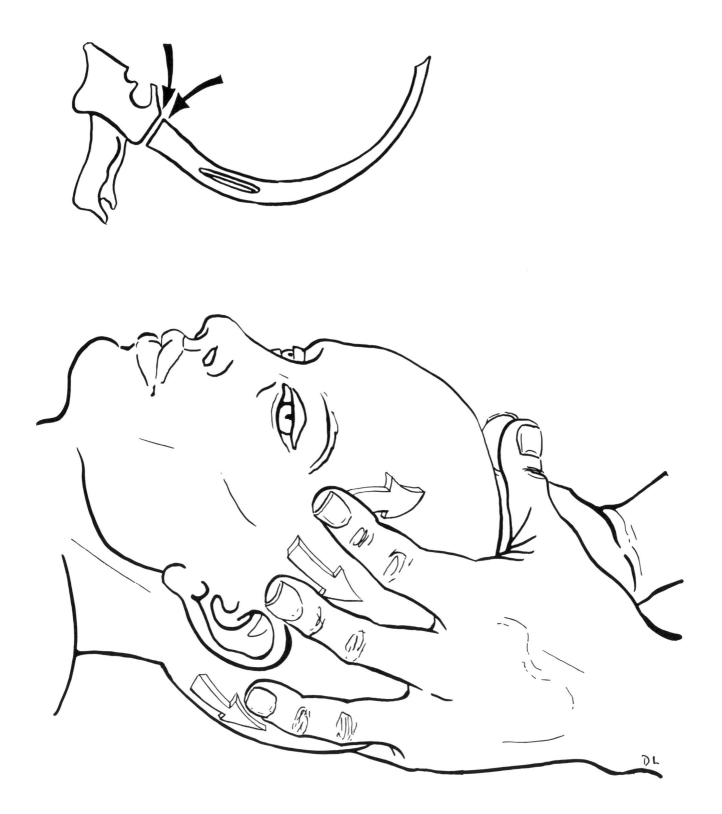

# EXTENSION MOVEMENT

## FRONTO-OCCIPITAL HOLD

### Objectives

- To assess the amount of inherent cranial motion during extension (and therefore during internal rotation).
- To directly correct a flexion lesion.
- To indirectly correct an extension lesion.
- To assess the freedom of motion of any particular cranial bone, within the context of cranial motion as a whole, during the relaxation phase of the cranial mechanism.

### Movement

Using the fronto-occipital hold (page 12), the practitioner proceeds in the following manner. During the relaxation phase of the cranial mechanism, the lower hand, under the occiput, moves the lateral angles cephalad in a circular movement around the transverse axis, while the upper hand simultaneously draws the greater wings of the sphenoid around the transverse axis in a cephalad and posterior direction.

### Comment

When the upper hand grips the greater wings of the sphenoid, the practitioner should avoid putting any pressure on the frontal bone which could induce a paradoxical movement.

When the upper hand has made its contacts behind the external orbital process of the frontal bone, it should execute the same movement as described above.

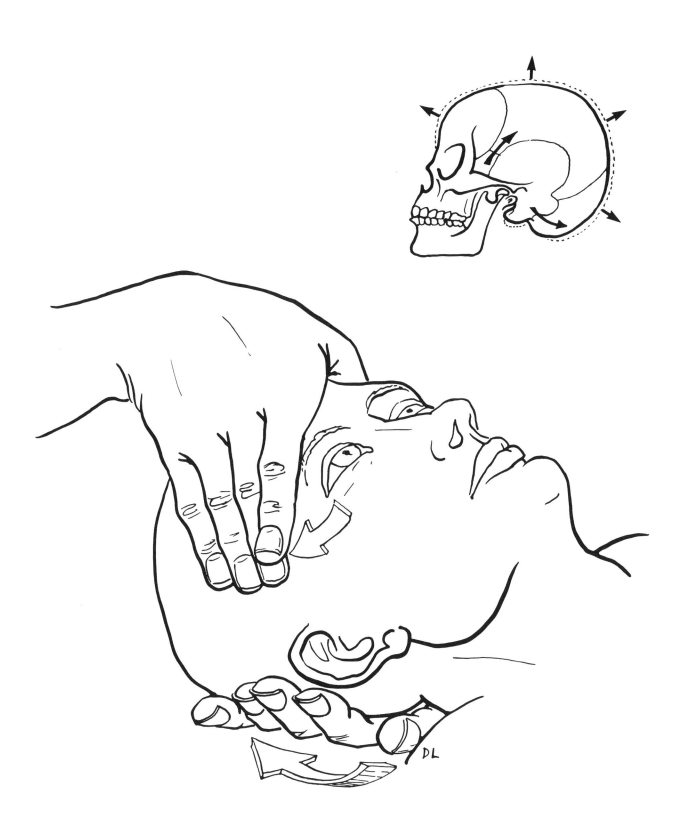

# TORSION MOVEMENT

## VAULT HOLD

**Objectives**

- To assess the amount of inherent cranial motion in torsion, during the cranial expansion phase.
- To directly correct an opposite torsion lesion, i.e., executing a torsion to the right to correct a lesion on the left.
- To indirectly reduce a torsion lesion on the corresponding side.
- To assess the freedom of motion of any particular cranial bone, within the physiological adaptive movement of torsion, during the expansion phase of the cranial mechanism.

**Movement** (torsion to the right)

Using the vault hold (page 10), the practitioner proceeds in the following manner. During the expansion phase of the cranial mechanism, the practitioner's right index finger draws the greater wing of the sphenoid (or the right external orbital process of the frontal bone) cephalad, while the left ring finger moves the left lateral angle of the occiput cephalad.

If this is not being used as a corrective technique, the practitioner should permit the mechanism to return to its inherent motion after having followed the mechanism toward the right torsion.

**Comment**

Each of the elements of this maneuver must be perfectly coordinated. In this technique, both flexion and torsion occur during the expansion phase.

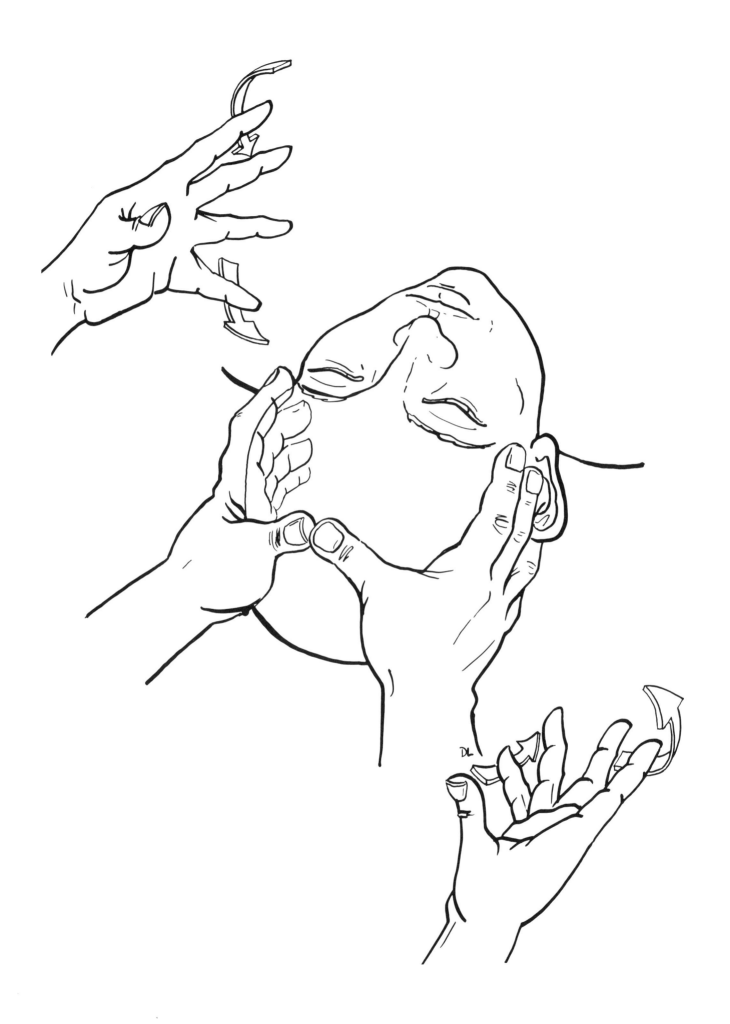

# TORSION MOVEMENT

## FRONTO-OCCIPITAL HOLD

**Objectives**

- To assess the amount of inherent cranial motion in torsion, during the cranial expansion phase.
- To directly correct an opposite torsion lesion, i.e., executing a torsion to the right to correct a lesion on the left.
- To indirectly reduce a torsion lesion on the corresponding side.
- To assess the freedom of motion of any particular cranial bone, within the physiological adaptive movement of torsion, during the expansion phase of the cranial mechanism.

**Movement** (torsion to the right)

Using the fronto-occipital hold (page 12), the practitioner, seated on the side opposite the torsion, proceeds in the following manner. During the expansion phase, the practitioner adds the torsion component to the usual flexion movement.

Upper hand: the middle finger elevates the right greater wing of the sphenoid in a cephalad direction around the anteroposterior glabella-inion axis, the practitioner's forearm pronating slightly. The thumb accompanies the movement of the left greater wing.

Lower hand: this hand elevates the left lateral angle of the occiput (or the posteroinferior angle of the left parietal) around the same anteroposterior axis. The forearm on that same side also pronates slightly.

During the relaxation phase of the cranial motion the practitioner is passive, initiating no action at the points of contact, but merely following the motion.

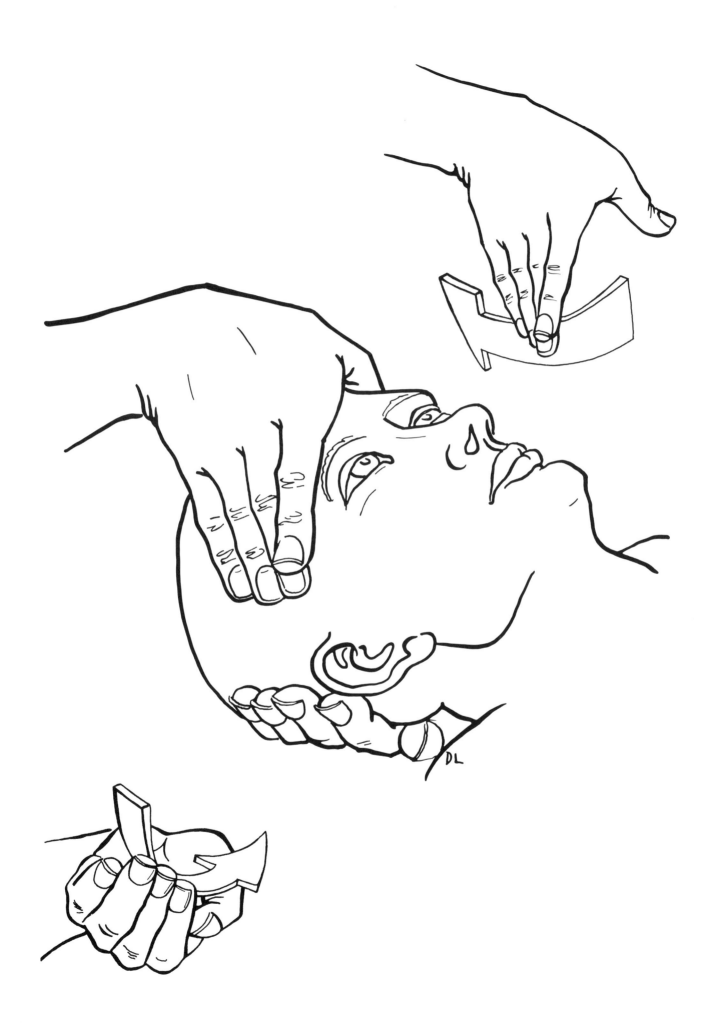

# SIDE BENDING ROTATION MOVEMENT

## VAULT HOLD

**Objectives**

- To assess the amount of side bending rotation motion during the expansion phase of the cranial mechanism.

- To directly correct a side bending rotation lesion of the opposite direction, i.e., a right side bending rotation will directly correct a left side bending rotation.

- To indirectly treat a side bending rotation lesion located on the same side.

- To assess the freedom of motion of any particular cranial bone, within the physiological adaptive movement of side bending rotation, during the expansion phase of the cranial mechanism.

**Movement** (right side bending rotation)

Using the vault hold (page 10), the practitioner proceeds as follows.

To execute a side bending rotation on the right, only the left hand is active, inducing the movement. The right hand, which is passive, monitors the proper development of this movement on the right side of the cranium.

During the expansion phase, the practitioner augments normal flexion while the side bending rotation movement is performed, as follows. All the fingers of the left hand (which are spread out without losing the points of contact) tend to draw nearer to one another. The practitioner pulls the left hand slightly cephalad along the longitudinal axis of the forearm. As the fingers of the right hand separate, they are allowed to move in a caudal direction.

During the relaxation phase of the cranial motion, the practitioner remains passive on the left as well as the right side.

**Comment**

The only possible difficulty in performing this action involves attaining optimum synchronization of the side bending rotation with normal flexion, and simultaneously with the expansion phase of cranial motion.

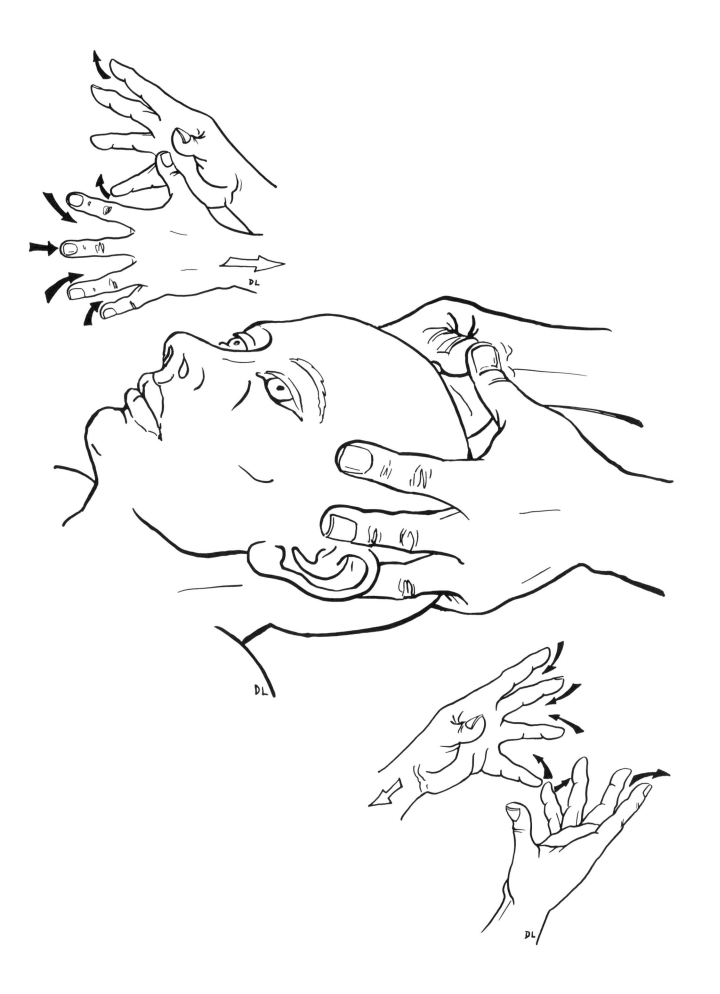

# SIDE BENDING ROTATION MOVEMENT

## FRONTO-OCCIPITAL HOLD

**Objectives**

- To assess the freedom of motion in the cranial mechanism during the side bending rotation movement.
- To directly correct a side bending rotation lesion on the opposite side.
- To indirectly treat a side bending rotation lesion on the same side.
- To assess the freedom of motion of any particular cranial bone, within the physiological adaptive movement of side bending rotation, during the expansion phase of the cranial mechanism.

**Movement** (right side bending rotation)

Using the fronto-occipital hold (page 12), the practitioner proceeds as follows.

During the cranial expansion phase, the practitioner adds a side bending rotation movement to the flexion in the following manner:

— around the two vertical axes of the sphenoid and occipital bones, both hands (while still gently maintaining their points of contact) draw closer together on the left side, and move apart on the right side;

— meanwhile, around the anteroposterior cranial axis, the hands move down toward the chin on the right, and up toward the vertex on the left.

The result is a well-rounded movement which draws the point of contact on the greater wing of the right sphenoid caudally, anteriorly and medially, while the right portion of the occiput moves caudally, posteriorly and medially.

During the relaxation phase of cranial motion, the practitioner allows the mechanism to return toward a neutral position.

**Comment**

The only possible difficulty in performing this action involves attaining optimum synchronization of the side bending rotation with normal flexion, and simultaneously with the expansion phase of cranial motion.

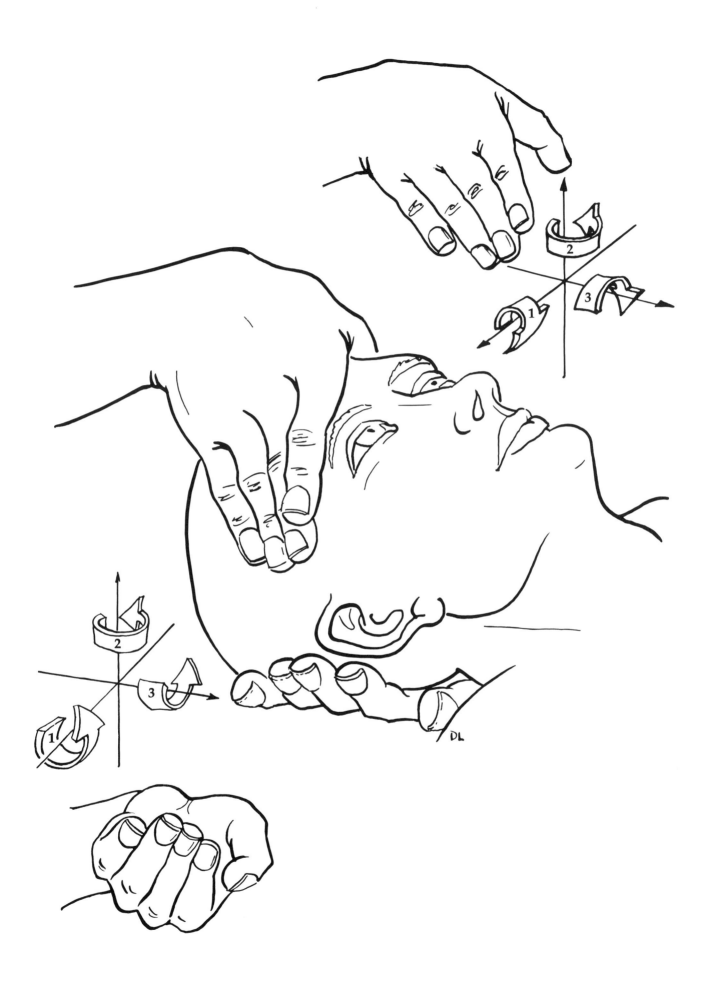

# LATERAL STRAINS OF THE CRANIAL BASE

## VAULT HOLD

### Objectives

- To assess the amount of motion in the cranial base during lateral movement induced by the practitioner's fingers.
- To reduce the tensions impeding the freedom of that motion, either directly or indirectly.
- To assess the freedom of motion of any particular cranial bone, within the context of cranial motion as a whole, during both the lateral movement induced by the practitioner's fingers, and during the expansion phase.

### Movement (right lateral strain)

This technique is performed by drawing the sphenoid and occiput in the same direction around their respective vertical axes.

Using the vault hold (page 10), the practitioner proceeds as follows.

During the expansion phase of cranial motion:

— on the right, the index finger draws the right greater wing of the sphenoid in a slightly anterior direction, while the ring and little fingers move the occiput in the same direction;

— on the left, the index finger draws the left greater wing of the sphenoid posteriorly, while the ring and middle fingers displace the occiput in the same direction.

During the relaxation phase of cranial motion, the inactive fingers maintain their points of contact, passively accompanying the cranial motion on its return to the neutral position.

### Comment

The direction of this maneuver is simply reversed at the finger level for a left lateral strain.

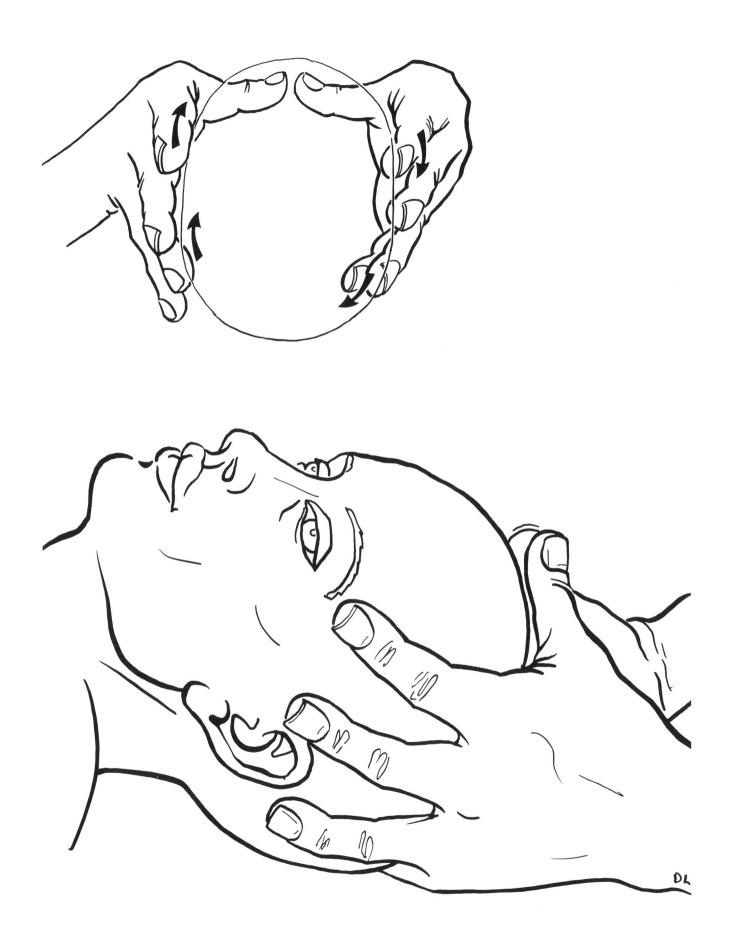

# LATERAL STRAINS OF THE CRANIAL BASE

## FRONTO-OCCIPITAL HOLD

**Objectives**

- To assess the amount of motion in the cranial base during a lateral movement induced by the practitioner's fingers.

- To reduce the tensions impeding freedom of that motion, either directly or indirectly.

- To assess the freedom of motion of any particular cranial bone, within the context of cranial motion as a whole, during both the lateral strain pattern induced by the practitioner's fingers and the expansion phase.

**Movement** (right lateral strain, practitioner sitting to the patient's left)

This technique is performed by drawing the sphenoid and occiput in the same direction around their respective vertical axes.

Using the fronto-occipital hold (page 12), the practitioner proceeds as follows. During the expansion phase of cranial motion the practitioner's upper hand draws the right greater wing of the sphenoid anteriorly, the forearm pronating slightly with the practitioner's thumb used as a firm base to maintain stability. The lower hand moves the right part of the occiput anteriorly, with the left forearm supinating very slightly.

During the relaxation phase, the practitioner's fingers simply accompany the motion back to the neutral position.

**Comment**

The direction of this maneuver is simply reversed at the finger level for a left lateral strain.

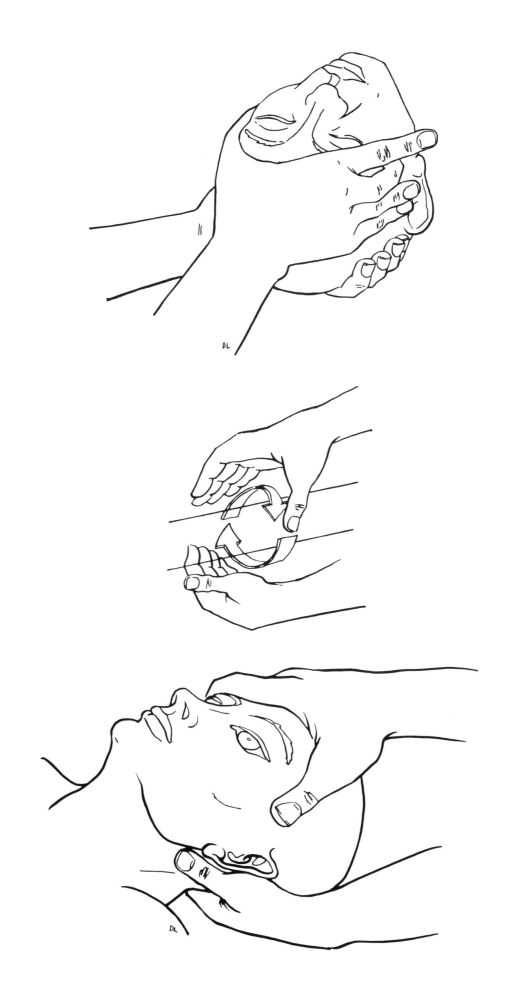

# VERTICAL STRAINS OF THE CRANIAL BASE

## VAULT HOLD

**Objectives**

- To assess the amount of motion in the cranial base during a vertical movement induced by the practitioner's fingers.

- To reduce the tensions impeding freedom of that motion, either directly or indirectly.

- To assess the freedom of motion of any particular cranial bone, within the context of cranial motion as a whole, when the vertical strain pattern induced by the practitioner's fingers occurs during the expansion phase of cranial motion.

**Movement** (superior vertical strain)

This technique is performed by drawing the sphenoid and occiput in the same direction around their respective transverse axes. This causes one bone to move in flexion, and the other in extension.

Using the vault hold (page 10), the practitioner proceeds as follows. During the expansion phase of cranial motion, the index fingers move the greater wings of the sphenoid in flexion (i.e., caudally and anteriorly), while the little fingers draw the occiput in extension (i.e., in a cephalad and posterior direction).

During the relaxation phase of cranial motion, the practitioner allows the cranial mechanism to return to the neutral position.

For an inferior vertical strain, the direction of this movement is simply reversed, i.e., the index fingers shift the greater wings of the sphenoid in extension, and the little fingers move the occiput in flexion.

**Comment**

The only possible difficulties with this maneuver involve coordinating the contrary movements of the index and little fingers.

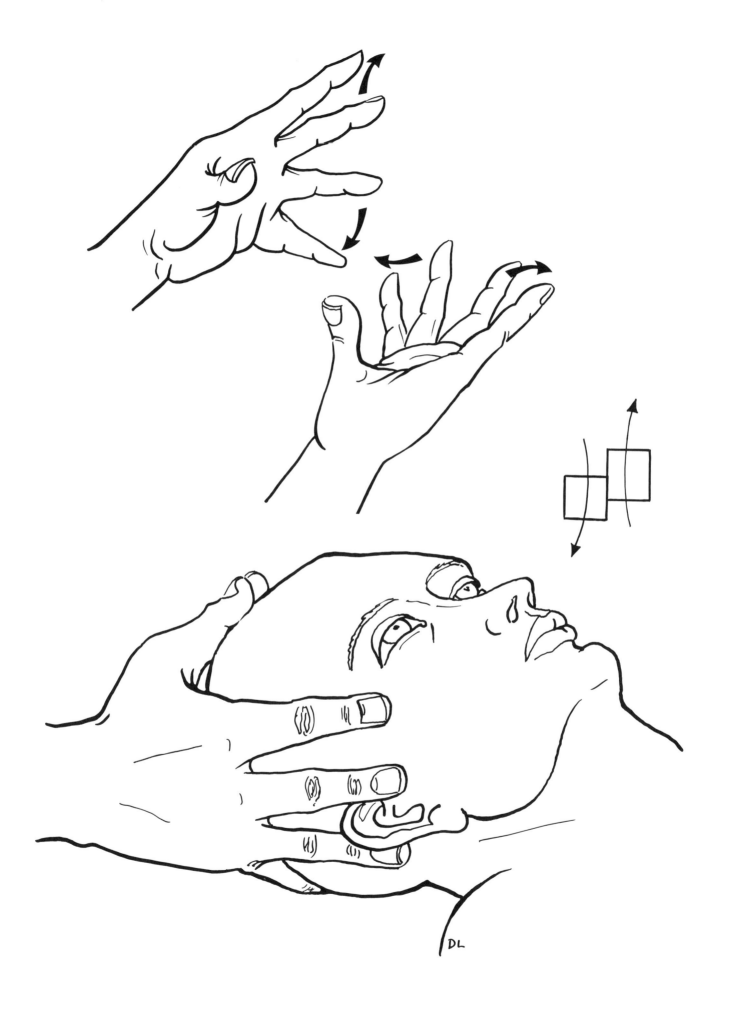

# VERTICAL STRAINS OF THE CRANIAL BASE

## FRONTO-OCCIPITAL HOLD

**Objectives**

- To assess the amount of motion in the cranial base during the vertical movement induced by the practitioner's fingers.
- To reduce the tensions impeding freedom of that motion, either directly or indirectly.
- To assess the freedom of motion of any particular cranial bone, within the context of cranial motion as a whole, when the vertical strain pattern induced by the practitioner's fingers occurs during the expansion phase of cranial motion.

**Movement** (superior vertical strain)

This technique is performed by drawing the sphenoid and occiput in the same direction around their respective transverse axes. This causes one bone to move in flexion, and the other to move in extension.

Using the fronto-occipital hold (page 12), the practitioner proceeds as follows. During the expansion phase of cranial motion, the practitioner's upper hand moves the sphenoid in flexion, and accompanies the greater wings of this bone anteriorly and caudally. In synchronization, the practitioner's lower hand draws the occiput in extension, i.e., posteriorly and cephalad.

During the relaxation phase of cranial motion, the practitioner allows the cranial mechanism to return to the neutral position.

For an inferior vertical strain, the direction of this movement is simply reversed: the upper hand moves the sphenoid in extension, while the lower hand draws the occiput in flexion.

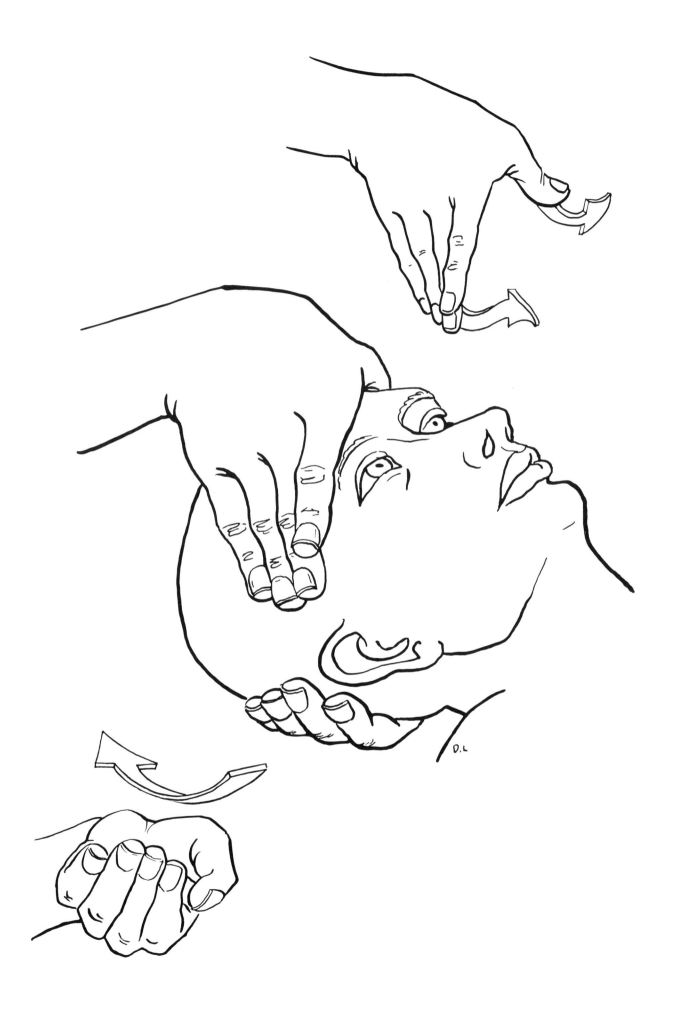

# DECOMPRESSION OF THE CRANIAL BASE

## VAULT HOLD

### Objective

To decompress the cranial base. Abnormal compression is indicated by assessing the ease of decompression, and also by such behavioral and subjective phenomena as the patient's lack of vitality, and depression.

### Movement

Using the vault hold (page 10), the practitioner proceeds as follows. During the expansion phase of cranial motion, the index fingers located on the greater wings of the sphenoid (or behind the external orbital processes of the frontal) tend to draw away from the little fingers (eventually reinforced by the ring fingers) placed on each side of the occipital bone.

The practitioner follows on the edge of this decompressive movement until a release is perceived. As the technique progresses, there will be accompanying twists and momentary halts as the various strain patterns of the particular patient come into play. These should be noted but not followed. It is important that the practitioner not let up on the decompressive force until the full release is perceived.

### Comment

This technique of decompression of the cranial base is most effective with children. The nature of the sphenobasilar joint, as well as the way in which forces are conducted from the periphery to the base, differs between children and adults. For adults, the technique by the fronto-occipital approach seems to be more effective.

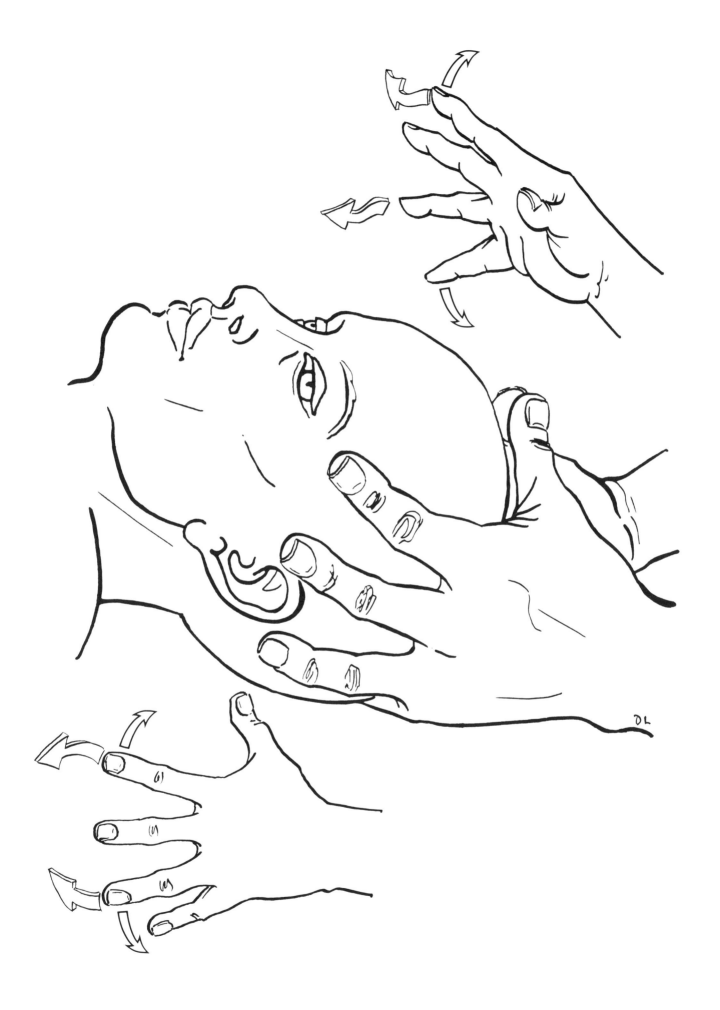

# DECOMPRESSION OF THE CRANIAL BASE

## FRONTO-OCCIPITAL HOLD

### Objective

To decompress the cranial base. Abnormal compression is indicated by assessing the ease of decompression, and also by such behavioral and subjective phenomena as the patient's lack of vitality, and depression.

### Movement

Using the fronto-occipital hold (page 12), the practitioner proceeds as follows. During the expansion phase of the cranial mechanism, the practitioner's upper hand will tend to move away from the lower hand. The latter rests on the top of the treatment table, cupping the occiput.

The practitioner follows on the edge of this decompressive movement until a release is perceived. As the technique progresses, there will be accompanying twists and momentary halts as the various strain patterns of the particular patient come into play. These should be noted but not followed. It is important that the practitioner not let up on the decompressive force until the full release is perceived.

It should be noted that the thumb and index finger (or middle finger) of the upper hand are placed either on the greater wings of the sphenoid, or behind the external orbital processes of the frontal bone.

### Comment

This approach is more appropriate for adults than children. Nevertheless, there may be obstacles to its proper realization, such as the patient's hair and occipital shape. It may then be necessary to employ the technique described on page 42.

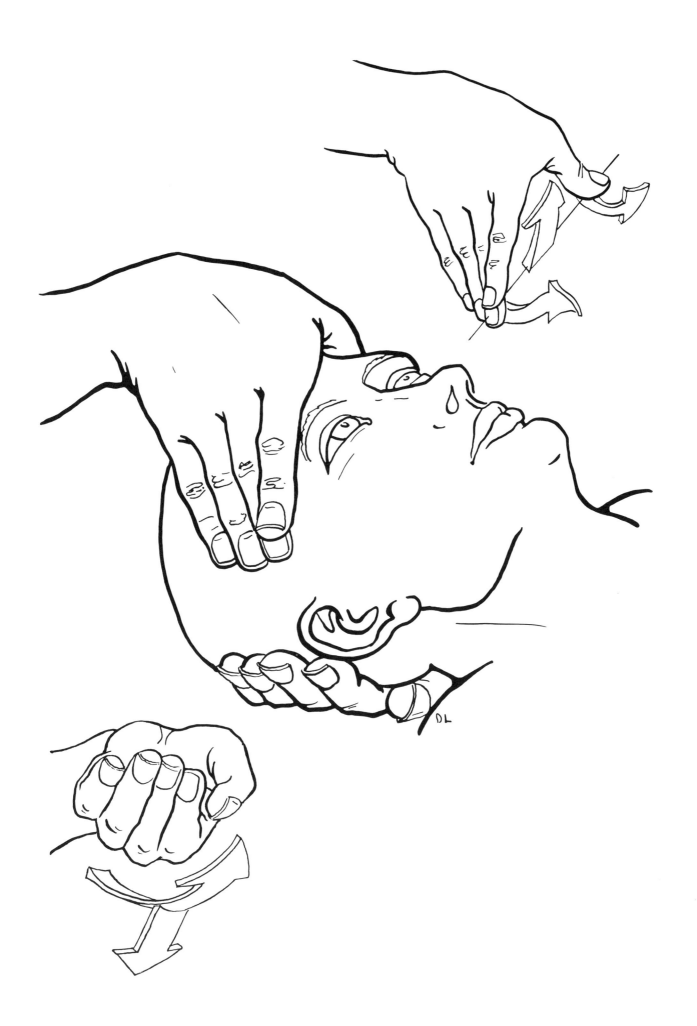

# DECOMPRESSION OF THE CRANIAL BASE

## TECHNIQUE FOR FOUR HANDS

### Objective

To decompress the cranial base when this cannot be accomplished by either of the two previous techniques.

### Position of the patient

Supine, comfortable and relaxed.

### Positions of the practitioners

This technique requires the presence of two practitioners working simultaneously in the following manner.

Practitioner A:

— at the patient's head;

— forearms and hands supine, fingers interlaced;

— contact with the thenar eminences at the external angles of the occipital squama, and thumbs on the mastoid processes of the temporal bones.

Practitioner B (who directs the maneuver):

— to one side of the patient, at the level of the patient's shoulders, the upper part of the body bent slightly over the patient;

— forearms and hands prone, fingers interlaced;

— contact with the thenar eminences behind the external orbital processes of the frontal bone, and contact with the hypothenar eminences on the frontosphenoidal area (depending upon the shapes of the practitioner's hands and the patient's cranium).

### Movement

Practitioner A holds the patient's occiput in the cup of his or her hands, which are supported by the top of the treatment table. Simultaneously, Practitioner B draws the anterior part of the patient's cranium anteriorly between his or her hands.

The practitioners follow on the edge of this decompressive movement until a release is perceived. As the technique progresses, there will be accompanying twists and momentary halts as the various strain patterns of the particular patient come into play. These should be noted but not followed. It is important that the practitioners not let up on the decompressive force until the full release is perceived.

### Comment

Besides requiring two practitioners, this technique sometimes involves the added disadvantage of imperfect coordination between the practitioners. This technique is best suited for particularly recalcitrant compressions of the cranial base.

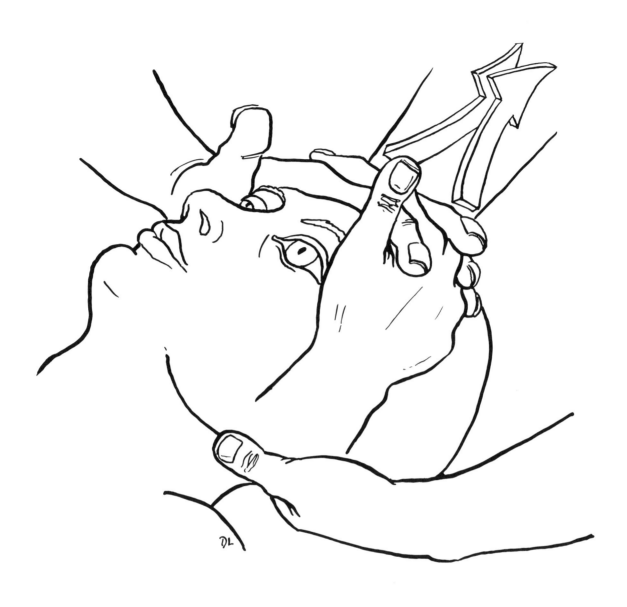

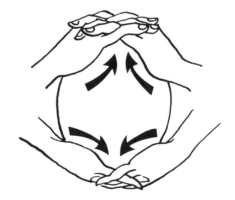

# SUTURAL OPENING TECHNIQUE

## Objective

This technique facilitates and enlarges the openings of all the sutures (especially at the vault level) with the exception of the temporoparietal and occipitomastoid sutures, which are compressed during the maneuver. It therefore allows the readjustment of the sutural system in general.

To experienced cranial practitioners, this technique affords an opportunity to determine whether temporal restrictions have their origins at the base or the vault.

## Position of the patient

Supine, comfortable and relaxed.

## Position of the practitioner

Seated at the patient's head, forearms resting on the treatment table which has been adjusted to a convenient height.

## Points of contact

The hands are supine, fingers interlaced, cupping the posterior part of the cranium so that the thenar eminences are situated at the mastoid portions of the temporal bones. The thumbs cover the superior part of the temporal bone, at the level of the temporoparietal suture, pointing toward the external orbital process of the frontal bone.

## Movement

This maneuver proceeds, with minutely increasing intensity, as follows.

1st phase:  the practitioner follows the cranial relaxation phase.

2nd phase:  by maintaining the same pressure, the expansion phase is impeded.

3rd phase:  the relaxation phase of the cranium is followed with very slight force.

4th phase:  an increase in pressure partly counteracts the ensuing expansion phase.

These phases are repeated until a general release is perceived.

## Comment

This technique should only be used by experienced practitioners, and then only when the situation demands. Whenever it is used, it is mandatory that it be followed by techniques to balance the temporoparietal and occipitomastoid areas. In order for this technique to be effective, it must be carried out for several cycles of the cranial mechanism.

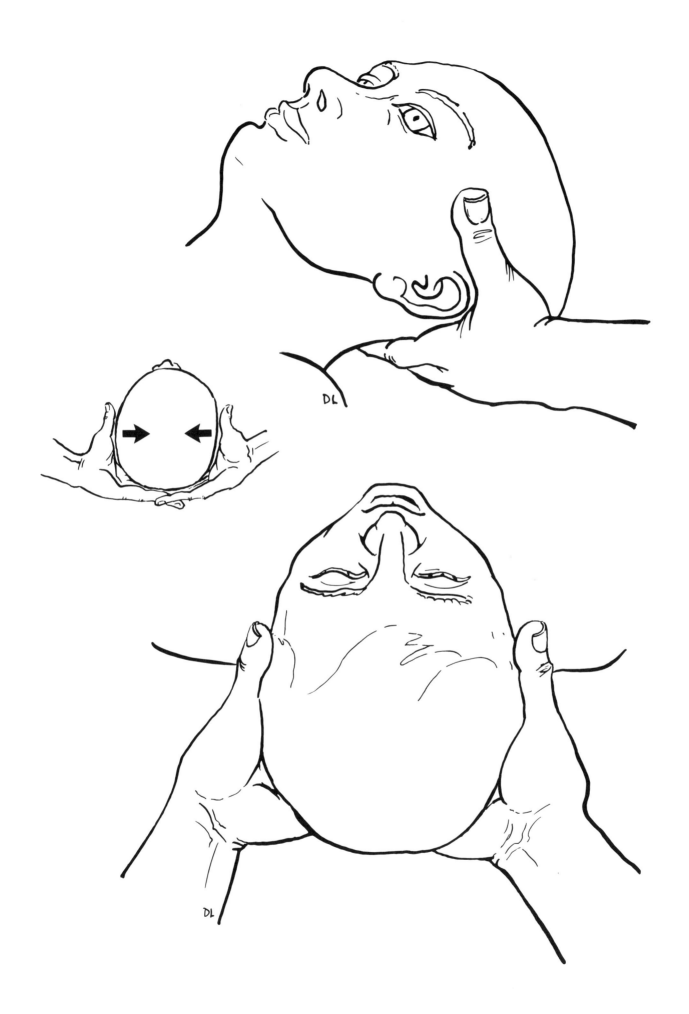

# COMPRESSION OF THE FOURTH VENTRICLE

**Objectives**

- Most commonly, to bring about a general relaxation of the patient. For this reason a cranial treatment will often start with this technique for patients who are ill-at-ease.

- As a general technique, to enhance the motion of the cranial rhythmic impulse.

**Position of the patient**

Supine, comfortable and relaxed.

**Position of the practitioner**

Seated at the patient's head, forearms resting on the treatment table which has been adjusted to a convenient height.

**Points of contact**

The practitioner closes his hands under the occiput, with fingers intertwined so as to form a hollow in which the occipital squama is held. The practitioner's thenar eminences are placed laterally to the external occipital protuberance, and medially to the lateral angles of the occipital squama.

**Movement**

During the relaxation phase, the practitioner exerts, with the deep flexor muscles of the fingers, a gentle, progressive and continuous pressure medially and cephalad. This has the effect of promoting extension and slightly increasing the anterior concavity of the patient's occipital squama. The pressure is maintained until a release is perceived, together with a sense of softening and warmth in the occiput. This is often accompanied by slight sweating, deep sighing and/or slow and deep breathing of the patient.

In an acceptable variation, this maneuver is executed rhythmically in exact synchronization with the pulmonary respiration. The practitioner encourages extension when the patient exhales, and relaxes his or her hands when the patient inhales. This process is continued until a release is perceived.

**Comment**

This maneuver must be avoided with any patient having recent cranial trauma, cerebral hemorrhage, other cerebrovascular accidents of recent onset or malignant hypertension.

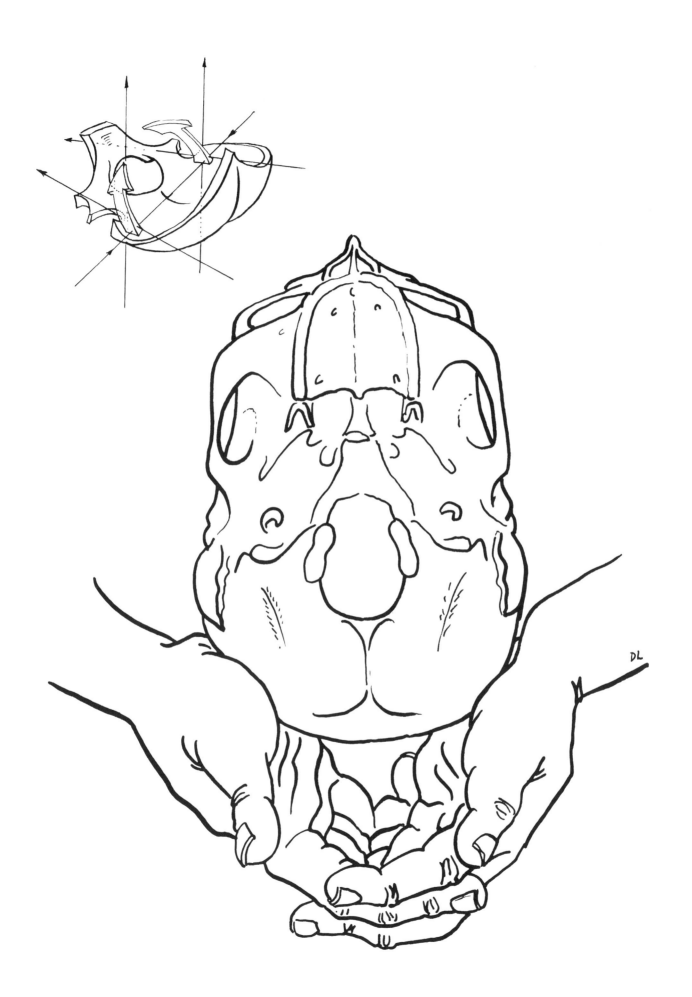

# ALTERNATING ROTATION OF THE TEMPORALS

## Objectives

- To normalize the lateral expansion of the cranium.
- To temporarily reduce (or, less frequently, to increase) the frequency of the cranial rhythmic impulse.
- To restore the balance of the cranial mechanism when it has been disturbed for any reason, including improper treatment. This technique has a calming effect; accordingly, many practitioners conclude their treatments with it.

## Position of the patient

Supine, comfortable and relaxed.

## Position of the practitioner

Seated at the patient's head, forearms resting on the treatment table which has been adjusted to a convenient height.

## Points of contact

The practitioner's hands are supine, with fingers intertwined. The hands cup the upper cervical spine and the occipital squama. Thumbs are placed parallel to the anterior border of the mastoid processes. The thenar eminences contact the corresponding mastoid portions of the temporal.

## Movement

The alternating movement is induced solely by the index or middle fingers, which are crossed at the second metacarpal joint. The other fingers simply follow the movement.

The practitioner alternately rolls one index finger on top of the other (or a middle finger on top of the other) at the second joint, which acts as a pivot. The passive thumbs move in an arc, taking the temporals with them.

## Mode of operation

If stimulation is the objective, the frequency (or amplitude) of the movement is very gradually increased.

If relaxation is the objective, the course of each phase is gradually reduced until movement is almost imperceptible. This is continued until a release is obtained. This approach is the most widely used at the conclusion of a cranial treatment.

## Comment

This technique is very easily performed. Nonetheless, the left-right balance of the hands is sometimes difficult for the poorly coordinated practitioner.

It is very important that a symmetrical balance of temporal motion be restored at the conclusion of this technique.

48

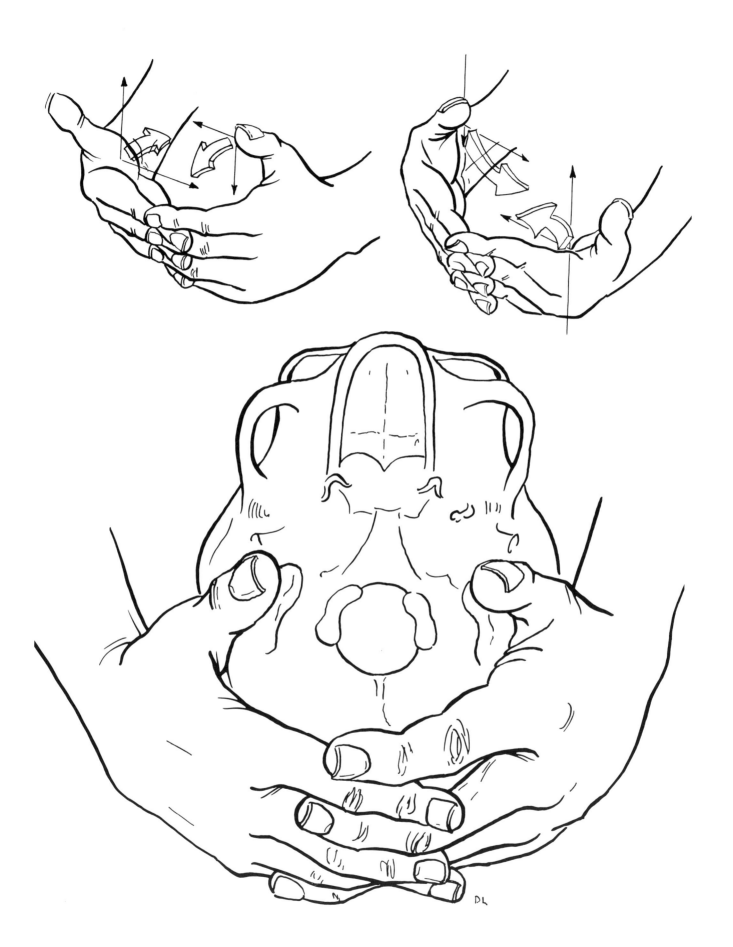

# SYNCHRONOUS ROTATION OF THE TEMPORALS

**Objective**

To provide a physiological stimulation of the cranial mechanism by increasing both its amplitude and rhythm.

**Position of the patient**

Supine, comfortable and relaxed.

**Position of the practitioner**

Seated at the patient's head, forearms resting on the treatment table which has been adjusted to a convenient height.

**Points of contact**

The practitioner's hands are supine, fingers interlaced, cupping the occipital squama. The practitioner places the thumbs parallel to the anterior border of the mastoid processes, the thenar eminences touching the corresponding mastoid portions.

**Movement**

Movement is generated by the deep flexor muscles of the fingers.

During the expansion phase of cranial motion, the tips of the practitioner's thumbs exert, on the top of the mastoid processes, a gentle pressure which is progressive and constant, moving medially and posteriorly.

During the relaxation phase, the practitioner progressively relaxes the pressure. He or she can, nevertheless, increase the amplitude of this phase by exerting pressure with the thenar eminences on the mastoid portions, medially and posteriorly.

The amplitude of the movement is then increased in both phases of cranial motion.

If desired, an increase in the frequency of cranial motion can easily be obtained by gradually increasing the rate of the maneuver.

**Comment**

While utilizing the mastoid lever, the practitioner must be very careful to respect the cranial articular physiology. Acceleration of the rhythm or increasing the amplitude of the motion should only be done very gradually.

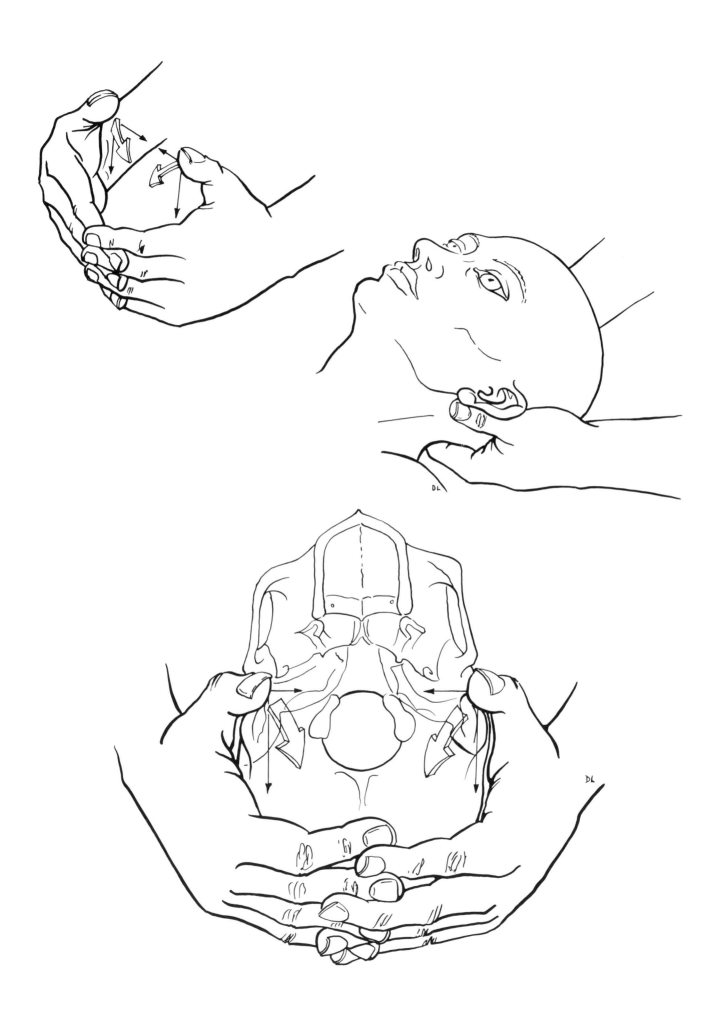

# REANIMATION TECHNIQUE

## "FATHER TOM"

### Objective

To restart the cranial mechanism's motion in cases of serious shock involving the peril of death (e.g., drowning or other cases of respiratory arrest) by a forced stimulation of the temporals in external rotation (maintenance of the expansion phase).

### Position of the patient

Supine.

### Position of the practitioner

At the patient's head, knees bent if the patient is lying on the ground.

### Points of contact

The practitioner's hands are joined under the occiput, fingers interlaced. The thumbs are placed along the mastoid processes of the temporal bones, the thenar eminences on the mastoid portions of the temporals.

### Movement

This technique must be applied vigorously, and is the ONLY exception to the rule of gentleness in cranial therapy.

The practitioner initiates a strong and simultaneous external rotation of both temporals by exerting a continuous posteromedial pressure on the mastoid processes. This pressure is maintained for a slow count of five, then released and repeated until a response occurs. The practitioner continues until a satisfactory rhythm and amplitude are obtained.

If the result is unsatisfactory after a few minutes, it is futile to continue.

### Comment

Because this technique is very powerful, it must only be applied in extreme situations, and then only by expert practitioners.

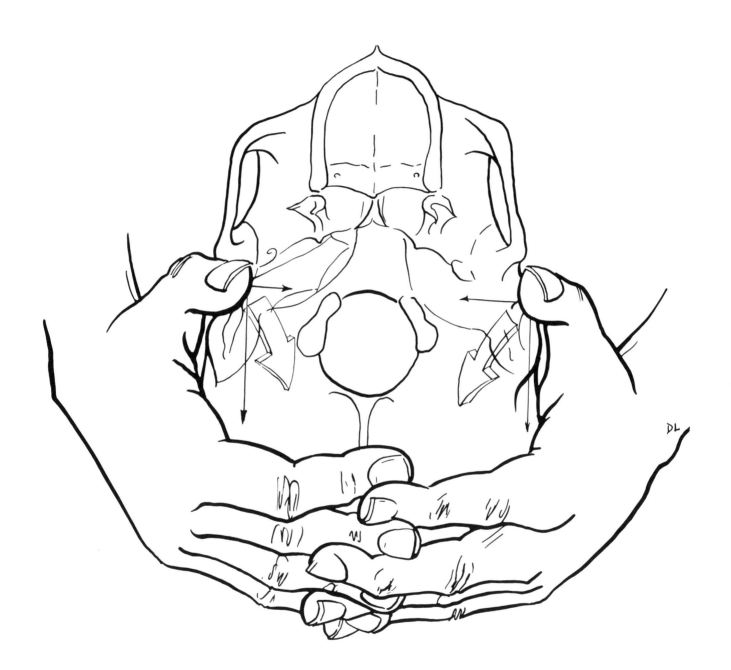

# GENERAL MOVEMENT OF THE CRANIUM

## CAUDAL INDEX FINGER INTRAORAL

### Objectives

- To restore sufficient amplitude to the motion of the cranial mechanism.
- To reestablish the normal rhythm of this motion.
- To reintegrate the specific motion of any particular bone into the general motion of the cranium.

### Position of the patient

Supine, comfortable and relaxed.

### Position of the practitioner

To one side of the patient, at his or her head.

### Points of contact

The cephalic hand holds the patient's occiput in the hollow of its palm. The axis of the forearm is in line with the longitudinal axis of the patient's body.

The index finger of the caudal hand touches the cruciate suture without pressure.

### Movement

During the expansion phase, the practitioner perfectly synchronizes the actions of both hands.

The cephalic hand increases the occipital flexion by accompanying this bone caudally and anteriorly, while the intraoral finger presses toward the patient's nostrils.

During the relaxation phase, the cephalic hand increases the occipital extension, drawing the latter cephalad and posteriorly, while the intraoral finger moves slightly back pressing on the cruciate suture in the direction of the root of the patient's nose.

In an acceptable variation, this technique can easily be applied when the patient is in a seated position. During the flexion of the occiput, the practitioner draws the patient's head anteriorly, on the passive index finger.

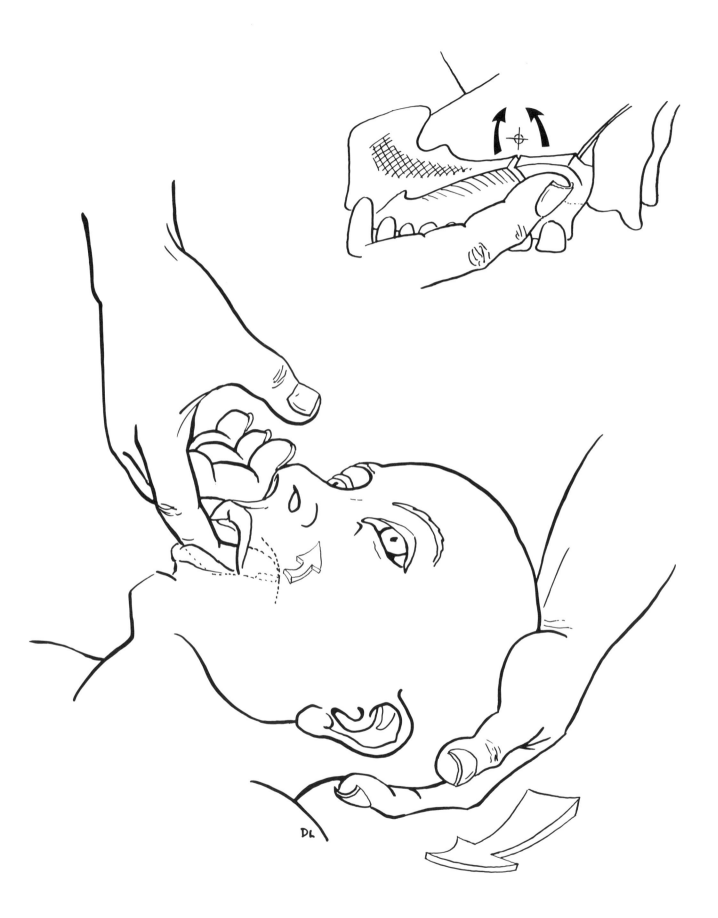

# OCCIPITAL PUMP

## Objectives

- First and foremost, to place the reciprocal tension membrane in equilibrium, especially at the occipital and temporal level.
- To obtain general relaxation (as with the compression of the fourth ventricle).
- To generate a return to normal after the occurrence of an improper cranial maneuver.

## Position of the patient

Supine, comfortable and relaxed.

## Position of the practitioner

Seated at the patient's head, forearms resting on the treatment table which has been adjusted to a convenient height.

## Points of contact

The practitioner places the pads of his or her index and middle fingers in the digastric grooves, behind the mastoid processes. The palms of the hands loosely cup the cranium; only their heels touch the parietal eminence area.

## Movement

After asking the patient to breathe slowly and deeply, the practitioner proceeds in the following manner.

1st phase:   the practitioner merely follows the two phases of cranial motion for a few cycles.

2nd phase:   the index and middle fingers initiate traction as soon as the relaxation phase begins.

3rd phase:   the index and middle fingers initiate an outward traction during the relaxation phase.

During the expansion phase, the practitioner gently maintains the outward traction.

Each of these phases develop over several cycles.

## Comment

This maneuver, which contains elements contrary to the generally accepted principles of cranial biomechanics, should always be followed by regularizing techniques, such as compression of the fourth ventricle (page 46), or alternating rotation of the temporals (page 48).

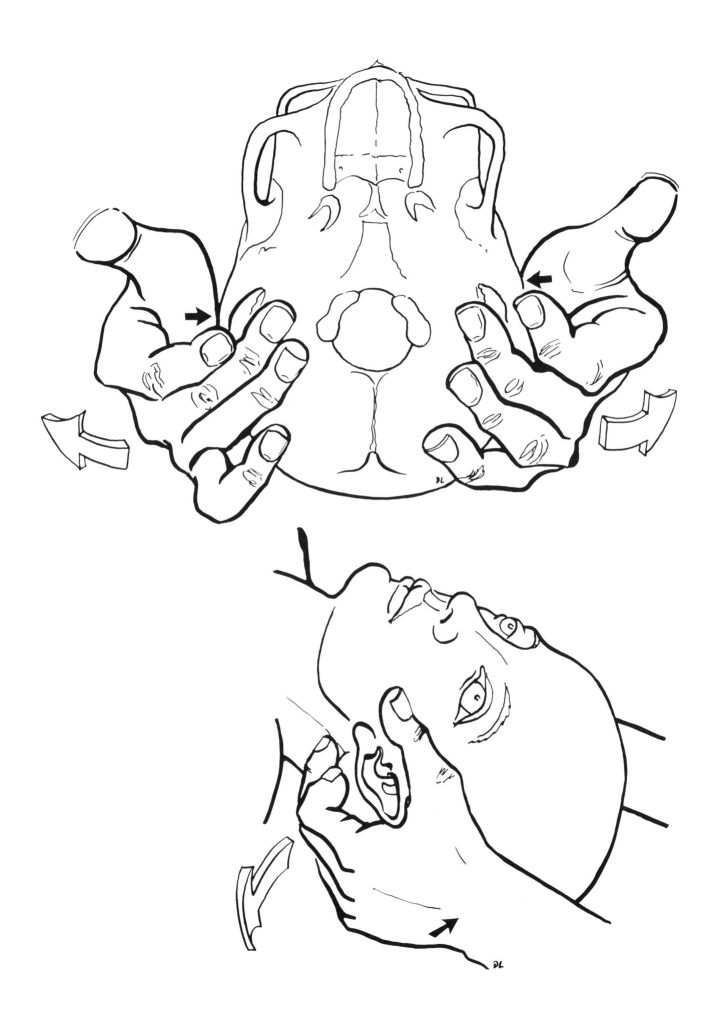

# SPREAD

## DIRECT CORRECTION

The spread is a type of procedure which can be adapted to any cranial technique using the expansion produced by the patient's body.

In direct correction, the practitioner manually follows exactly the opposite course taken by the lesional force.

For example, if the practitioner is performing a correction of right torsion lesion with a vault hold, he or she would proceed as follows. (The objectives, positions of patient and practitioner, and points of contact are all identical to those described for the vault hold on page 10.)

### Movement

During the expansion phase, the practitioner draws the right greater wing of the sphenoid posteriorly and caudally with the right index finger, while the left ring finger moves the posterior inferior angle of the left parietal (or the left lateral angle of the occiput) cephalad and caudally, following the mechanism to the point of balanced tension. This is maintained quietly and without strain, until the mechanism comes to a stop.

The patient is then asked to dorsiflex his or her left ankle and hold it steady. The practitioner at that time perceives a wave coming toward the point of balanced tension. After a short period of time (a few seconds to a few minutes), a wobbling motion and/or pulsation is perceived. There is then a significant release that develops into a new point of balance of the cranium and a return to a rhythmic cadence of the cranial mechanism, with an increase in the freedom of movement. The patient relaxes the dorsiflexion of the left ankle, and the practitioner monitors the motion of the cranial mechanism for a few more cycles.

### Comment

The longest diagonal is always used, i.e., for problems with the right side of the head the left foot is dorsiflexed. For midline problems, both feet are dorsiflexed.

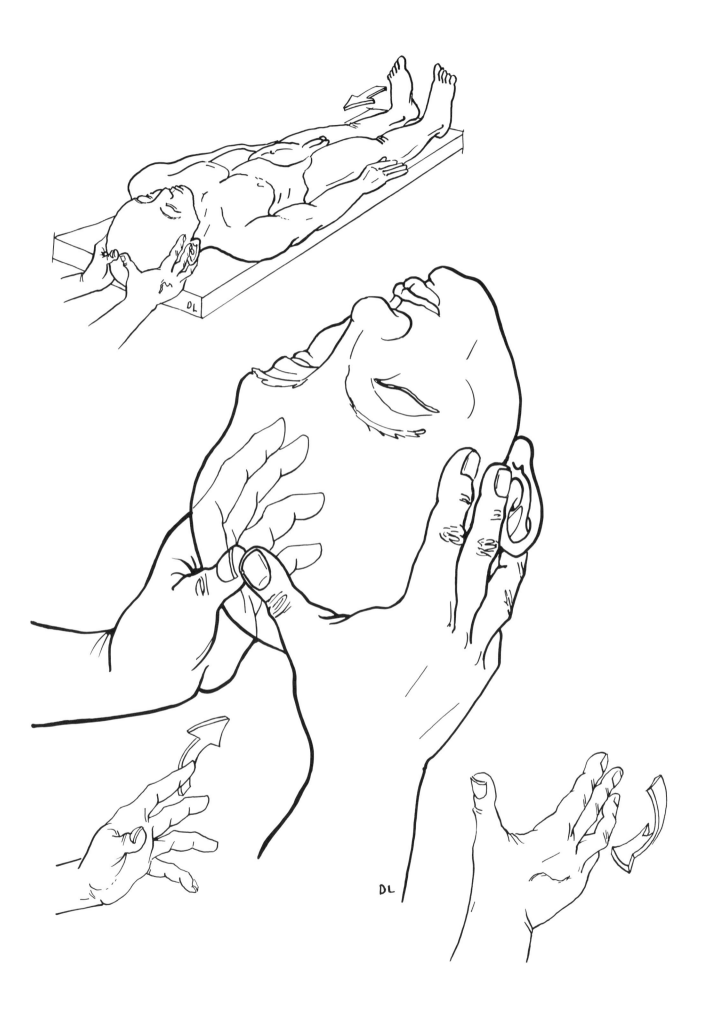

# SPREAD

## INDIRECT CORRECTION

The spread is a type of procedure which can be adapted to any cranial technique using the expansion produced by the patient's body.

In indirect correction, the practitioner follows the lesion pattern as far as it will go. This balances the reciprocal tension membrane, and allows the cranial motion to be fulfilled.

For example, if the practitioner is performing a correction of right torsion lesion with a vault hold, he or she would proceed as follows. (The objectives, positions of patient and practitioner, and points of contact are all identical to those described for the vault hold on page 10.)

### Movement

During the expansion phase, the practitioner draws the right greater wing of the sphenoid anteriorly and cephalad with the right index finger, while the left ring finger moves the posterior inferior angle of the left parietal (or the left lateral angle of the occiput) cephalad and caudally, following the mechanism to the point of balanced tension in the right torsion strain pattern. This is maintained quietly and without strain, until the mechanism comes to a stop.

The patient is then asked to dorsiflex his or her left ankle and hold it steady. The practitioner at that time perceives a wave coming toward the point of balanced tension. After a short period of time (a few seconds to a few minutes), a wobbling motion and/or pulsation is perceived. There is then a significant release that develops into a new point of balance of the cranium and a return to a rhythmic cadence of the cranial mechanism, with an increase in the freedom of movement. The patient relaxes the dorsiflexion of the left ankle, and the practitioner monitors the motion of the cranial mechanism for a few more cycles.

### Comment

The longest diagonal is always used, i.e., for problems with the right side of the head the left foot is dorsiflexed. For midline problems, both feet are dorsiflexed.

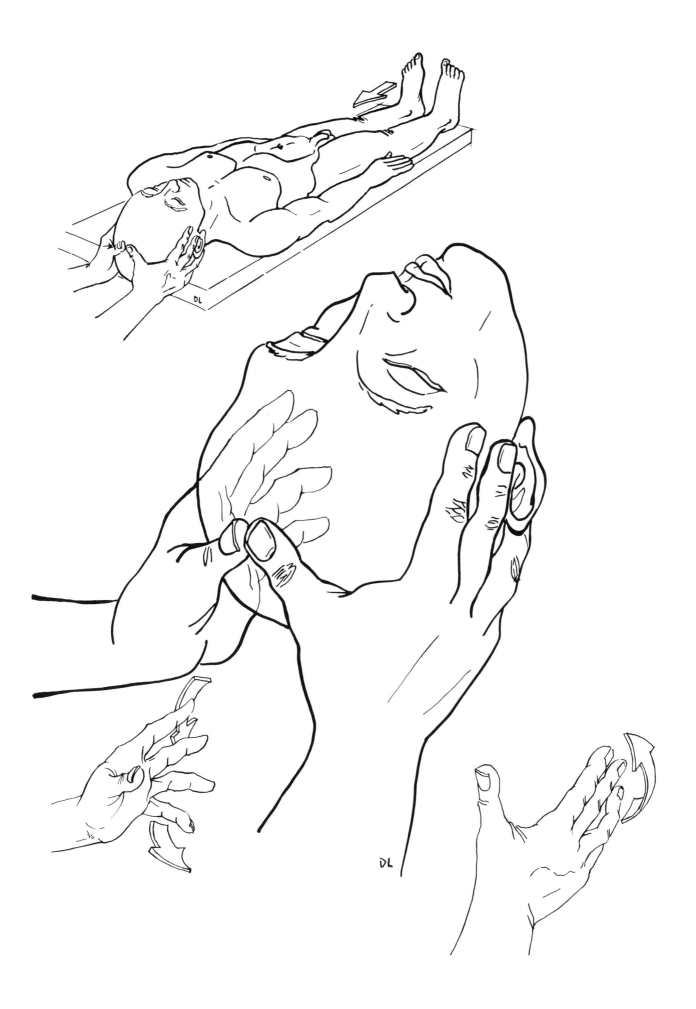

# SUTURAL SPREAD

## SUTURAL OPENING

### Objective

To take advantage of the opportunity afforded by the spread technique to open a cranial suture.

### Position of the patient

Supine, comfortable and relaxed.

### Position of the practitioner

Determined by the suture which is to be released.

The practitioner adjusts the table so that the patient's head is level with his or her hands.

### Points of contact

Two fingers of one hand, generally the middle and index fingers, are placed on the two edges of the sutural restriction. These contacts are gently made by the pads of the terminal phalanges.

One finger of the other hand, touching an opposite point of the cranium, forms the largest diagonal which separates it from the two fingers of the first hand.

### Movement

During the expansion phase, the fingers which are on the edges of the suture both draw slowly apart and maintain their divergence. The other finger, pointing in their direction, presses slightly on the cranial surface. This action is stopped only when the two opposite fingers perceive a release in the local tissues.

### Comment

This technique is variously known as the "V-spread," the direction of fluid technique, and the direction of energy technique.

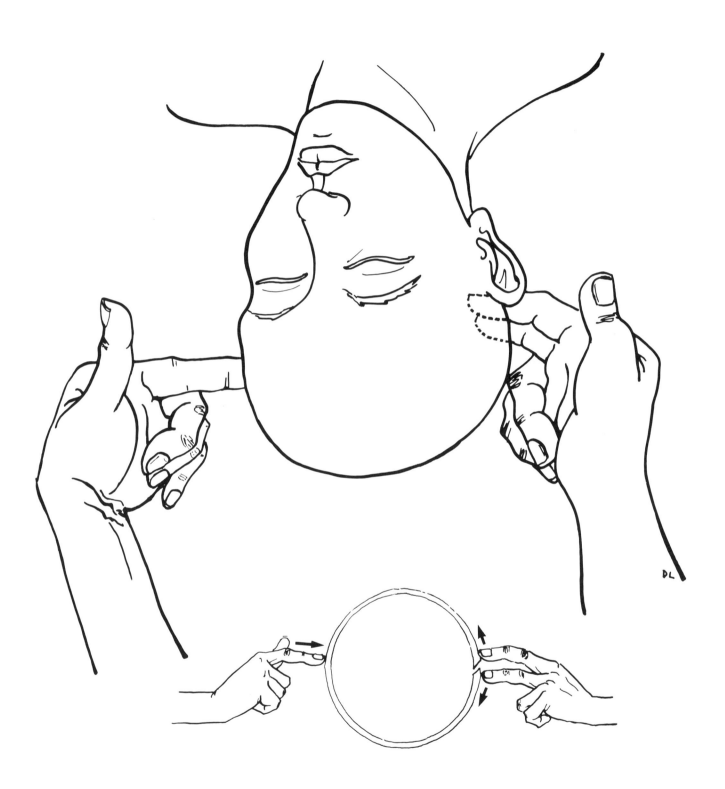

# II  Occipital Techniques

# OCCIPITOATLANTOID TEST

### Objectives

- To assess the freedom of motion of the craniovertebral junction, unilaterally or bilaterally.
- To cause a release of the tensions of the pariarticular occipitoatlantoid soft tissues.

### Position of the patient

Supine, comfortable and relaxed.

### Position of the practitioner

Seated at either side of the patient's head, the treatment table adjusted to a convenient height.

### Points of contact

The practitioner's caudal hand is perpendicular to the plane of the table and touches it with its ulnar aspect. The radial aspect of the index finger touches the musculature over the posterior arch of the atlas (which is released by the extension of the occipitoatlantoid joint). The cephalic hand holds the patient's forehead in its palm, between the anterior thumb and index finger.

### Movement

The cephalic hand alone is active. The caudal hand is used as a support and also to check the rate and assess the freedom of motion of the occipitoatlantoid articulation.

1st phase: the cephalic hand exerts a strictly vertical pressure along the plane of the supporting hand. This very gentle pressure is eased as soon as resistance is felt. This maneuver is repeated several times.

2nd phase: the practitioner then directs the pressure (still along the plane of the supporting hand) obliquely from right to left (right frontal to left mastoid). This maneuver checks the mobility of the left occipitoatlantoid articulation.

3rd phase: the practitioner exerts a comparable pressure from left to right to check mobility on the right side.

### Comment

If the pressure is held at the barrier until a release is perceived, this test can be converted into a treatment technique.

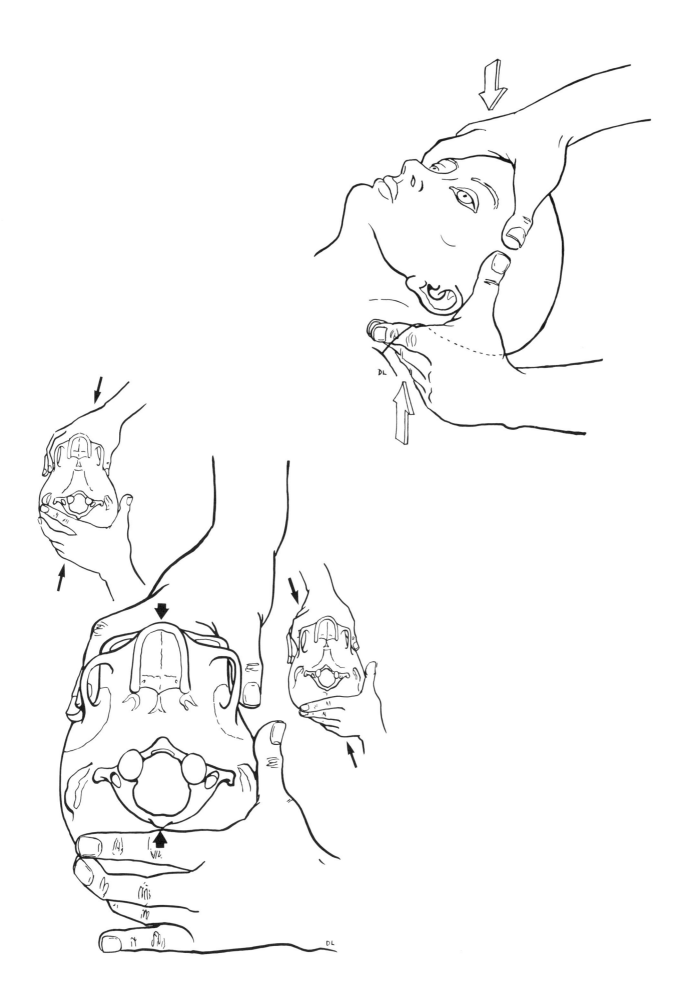

# EQUILIBRATION OF THE FORAMEN MAGNUM

## Objectives

- To free the suboccipital area of all the chronic tensions which affect it.
- To balance the foramen magnum area on the upper cervical spine at the conclusion of a cranial treatment, or following the application of occipital techniques.

## Position of the patient

Supine, comfortable and relaxed.

## Position of the practitioner

Seated at the patient's head, forearms resting on the treatment table which has been adjusted to a convenient height.

## Points of contact

The practitioner, with hands in a supine position, points the fingers in the direction of the ear on the opposite side of the patient's head. He or she slides the fingers under the occiput so that they are medial to the mastoid process. The thumbs, on the temporal bones, are used only to assess the balancing of the cranium.

## Movement

The following four phases must proceed smoothly.

1st phase:  the patient is asked to raise his or her head slightly. The head is rested on the practitioner's index and ring fingers.

2nd phase:  the free middle fingers palpate under the ridge on the inferior lateral aspect of the external occipital protuberance in search of increased tissue tension.

3rd phase:  when a sensitive zone is found, the practitioner leaves his or her middle finger on it. The other middle finger is placed on the corresponding spot on the other side. On the sensitive side, the patient's head is pulled slightly toward the practitioner. Finally, the practitioner rotates the patient's head toward the side opposite the lesion.

4th phase:  the practitioner maintains this new position until the release of the tension is perceived under the pad of the middle finger. The patient's head is then returned to its original position.

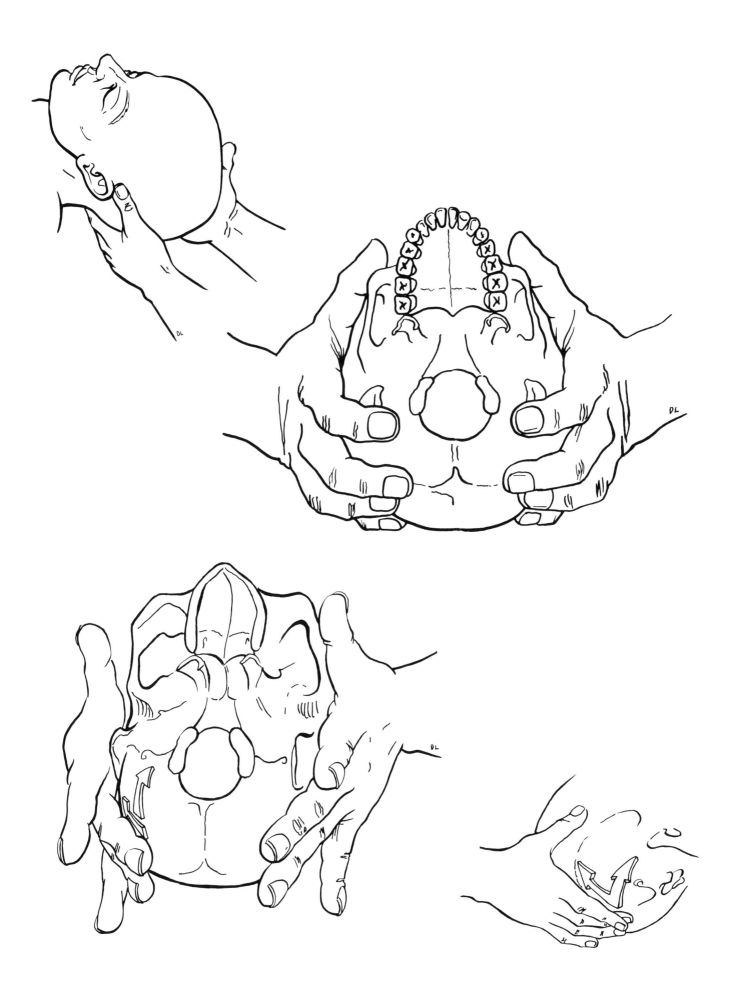

# ENLARGEMENT OF THE FORAMEN MAGNUM

### Objectives

- In adults, to release the tensions surrounding the foramen magnum as much as possible.
- In children, to indirectly draw apart the condylar masses of the occiput to the extent permitted by the flexibility of the bone. This "modelling" can only be carried out before the fusion of the squama and the two condylar portions (at the age of about seven or eight).

### Position of the patient

Supine, comfortable and relaxed.

### Position of the practitioner

Seated at the patient's head, forearms resting on the treatment table which has been adjusted to a convenient height.

### Points of contact

As in the previous technique, the practitioner tries to obtain a contact as near as possible to the foramen magnum. To this end, the pads of the index fingers penetrate, on both sides, the slight depression located between the two posterior and lateral muscular masses of the neck. The practitioner's forearms are supine, with the remaining fingers cupping the patient's cranium gently and with equal force.

### Movement

During the expansion phase, the practitioner (without losing contact) draws his or her index fingers apart, pulling them posteriorly, laterally and caudally. The palms follow the flexion motion.

During the relaxation phase, the traction is progressively eased. It is resumed during the next expansion phase. This process is continued until a release is perceived.

### Comments

This is a very effective treatment until the age of seven or eight, and is less effective after that age. This technique cannot be used in patients with "football players' neck," extremely hunched-up shoulders, or similar conditions.

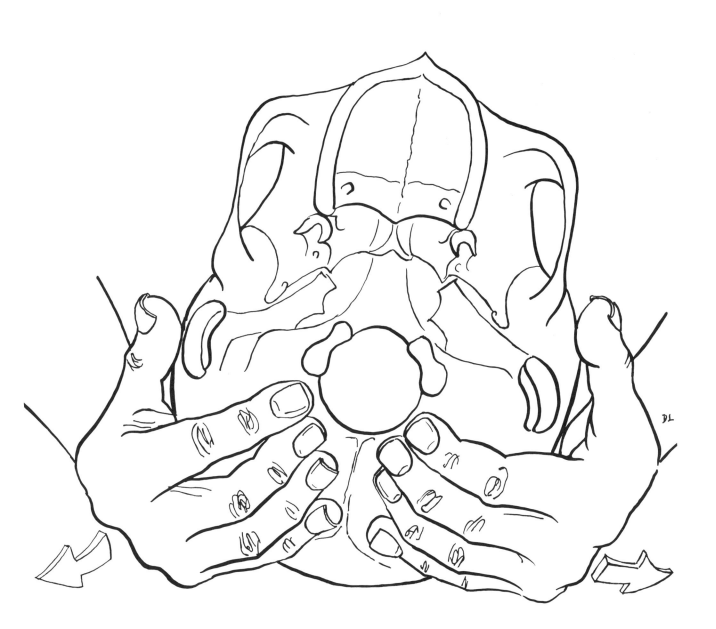

# OCCIPITOMASTOID OPENING

**Objective**

To release the occipitomastoid suture when there has been a traumatic lesion without true impaction.

**Position of the patient**

Supine, comfortable and relaxed.

**Position of the practitioner**

Seated at the patient's head, forearms resting on the treatment table which has been adjusted to a convenient height.

**Points of contact** (right occipitomastoid lesion)

The practitioner's left hand is supine and perpendicular to the longitudinal axis of the patient's body. It cups the occiput in its open palm. The tips of the fingers touch the right squamous angle, and the thumb touches the left angle.

The practitioner places the thumb of the right hand along the anterior border of the right mastoid process, with the thenar eminence positioned on the mastoid portion.

**Movement**

During the expansion phase, the practitioner's left hand increases the flexion of the occiput by drawing it caudally and anteriorly around its transverse axis. It is then rotated around its vertical axis to the left so as to open the right occipitomastoid suture.

Simultaneously, the tip of the thumb of the right hand exerts a gentle yet progressive and constant pressure, medially and posteriorly, on the tip of the right mastoid process.

During the ensuing phase, the practitioner eases the pressure from the right hand. To reinforce the action, this may be accompanied by pressure of the thenar eminence caudally and medially on the temporal mastoid portion. This process is continued until a release of the occipitomastoid suture is perceived.

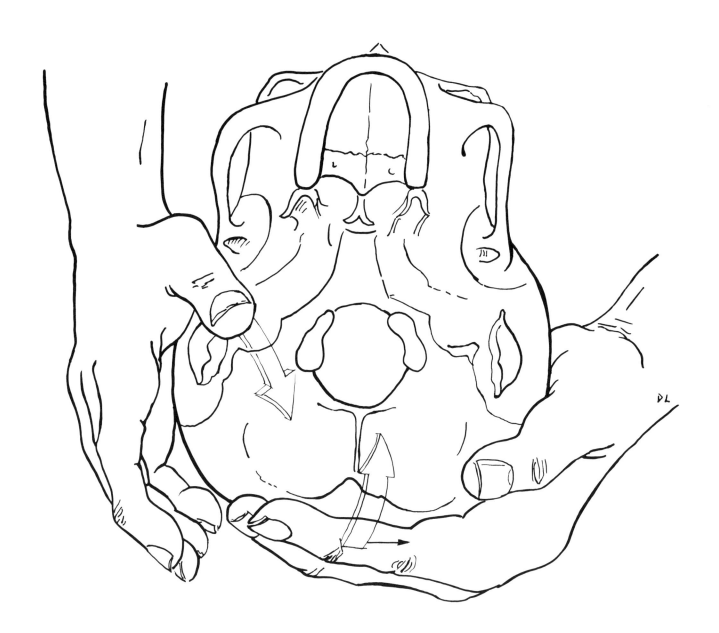

# OCCIPITOMASTOID DISIMPACTION

**Objective**

To free the occipitomastoid suture when there is a compression lesion, generally originating from trauma.

**Position of the patient**

Supine, comfortable and relaxed.

**Position of the practitioner**

Seated at the patient's head, forearms resting on the treatment table which has been adjusted to a convenient height.

**Points of contact**

The practitioner joins his or her hands under the occiput, fingers interlaced. Thumbs are placed along the mastoid processes of the temporals so that the thenar eminences touch the lateral angles of the occipital squama.

**Movement** (right occipitomastoid disimpaction)

The following five phases must proceed smoothly.

1st phase: during the relaxation phase, the practitioner increases pressure at the lateral angles of the occipital squama with the thenar eminences, as in compression of the fourth ventricle (page 46).

2nd phase: the practitioner draws the occiput posteriorly, disengaging it to the extent possible from the neighboring bones.

3rd phase: the practitioner widens the right sutural opening to the extent possible by a slight rotation of the occiput around its vertical axis, toward the left.

4th phase: during the expansion phase, while maintaining this sutural opening as wide as possible, the practitioner exerts a posterior and medial pressure with the right thumb on the tip of the right mastoid process.

5th phase: the practitioner only eases the pressure of the right thumb during the ensuing cranial phase. This cycle continues until disimpaction is achieved.

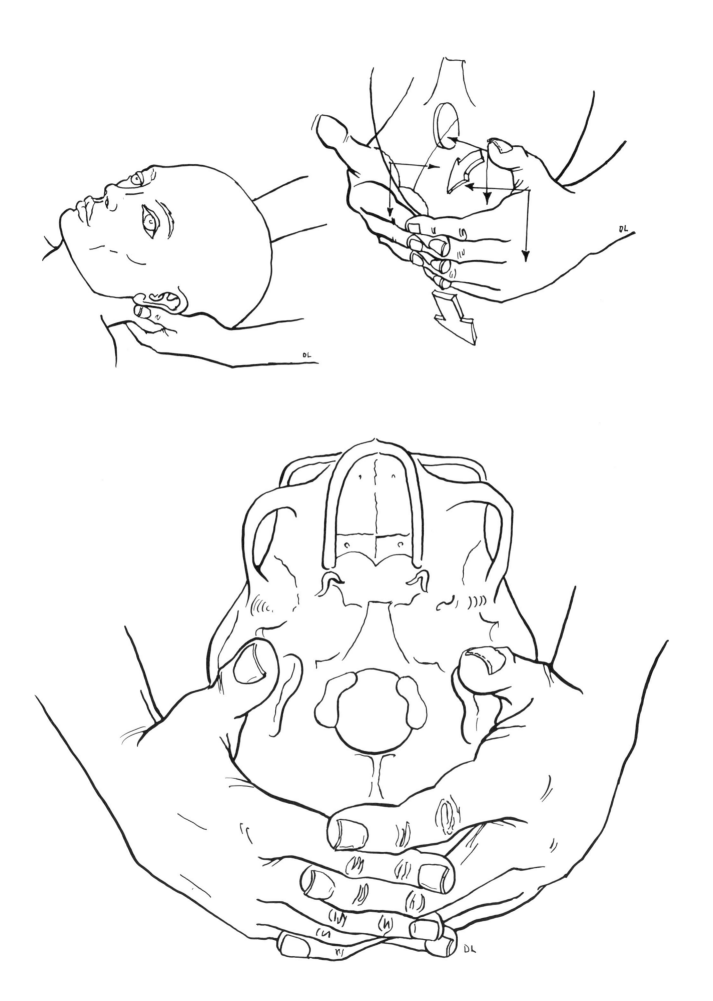

# TECHNIQUE FOR ANTERIOR OR POSTERIOR OCCIPUT

## Objective

To reduce unilateral, anterior or posterior lesions of the occipital bone around its vertical axis.

## Position of the patient

Supine, comfortable and relaxed.

## Position of the practitioner

Seated at the patient's head, forearms resting on the treatment table which has been adjusted to a convenient height.

## Points of contact

The practitioner interlaces his or her fingers so that they touch at the middle phalanx. The upper index finger is placed on the side of the lesion. The fingers are then supinated, exerting no pressure. The thumbs are horizontal and the thenar eminences cup the lateral angles of the patient's occipital squama. These are the only points of contact between the practitioner and the patient.

## Movement (lesion on the right)

Right anterior occiput: during the expansion phase, the practitioner pronates his or her hand, so that the right index finger rolls on the left one medially at the second joint.

The practitioner then resists the supinating effect on the index finger of the relaxation phase.

These two phases alternate during the application of the technique until a release is perceived.

Right posterior occiput: the order of the active and resisting phases is reversed. The practitioner supinates the right hand during the expansion phase by rolling the right index finger laterally against the left one.

## Comments

This technique must be repeated several times to be effective. It must be preceded by a release of the suture concerned.

Its performance requires that only one index finger be active.

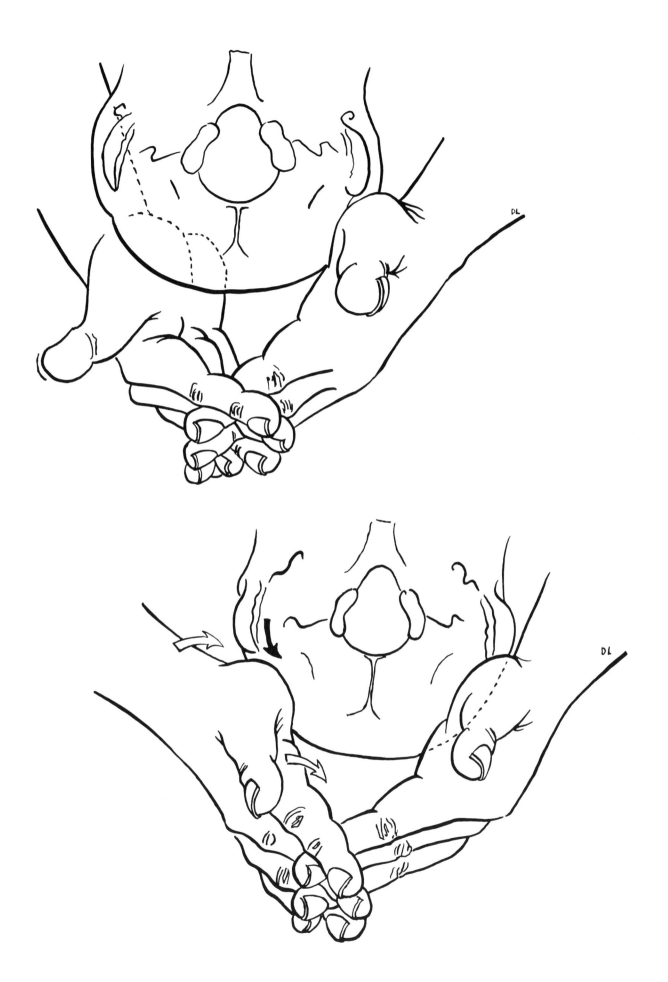

# REPOSITIONING OF THE OCCIPUT

**Objective**

The essential purpose of this technique is the complete repositioning of the occiput when it is the primary site of lesion. The other bones articulating with it (sphenoid, temporals and parietals) will then adjust themselves without difficulty.

**Position of the patient**

Supine, comfortable and relaxed.

**Position of the practitioner**

To one side of the patient's head.

**Points of contact**

The cephalic hand nestles the occipital squama in the concavity of its palm, following the longitudinal axis of the patient's body.

The thumb and index finger of the caudal hand control the sphenoid by its greater wings and envelop the frontal, while the pad of the little finger (intrabuccal) controls the pterygoid process on the opposite side.

**Movement**

The anterior aspect of the cranium is perfectly controlled by the hold of the caudal hand.

During the expansion phase, the practitioner positions the occiput in a state of balanced tension on its transverse and vertical axes.

During the relaxation phase, the practitioner gently resists the return to the neutral position.

The practitioner continues this process over several cycles until a release is perceived. This signals an integration of the occipital motion within the general motion of the cranium.

**Comment**

Either the vault hold (page 10) or the fronto-occipital hold (page 12) will allow the practitioner to assess the quality of this integration with the general motion of the cranium.

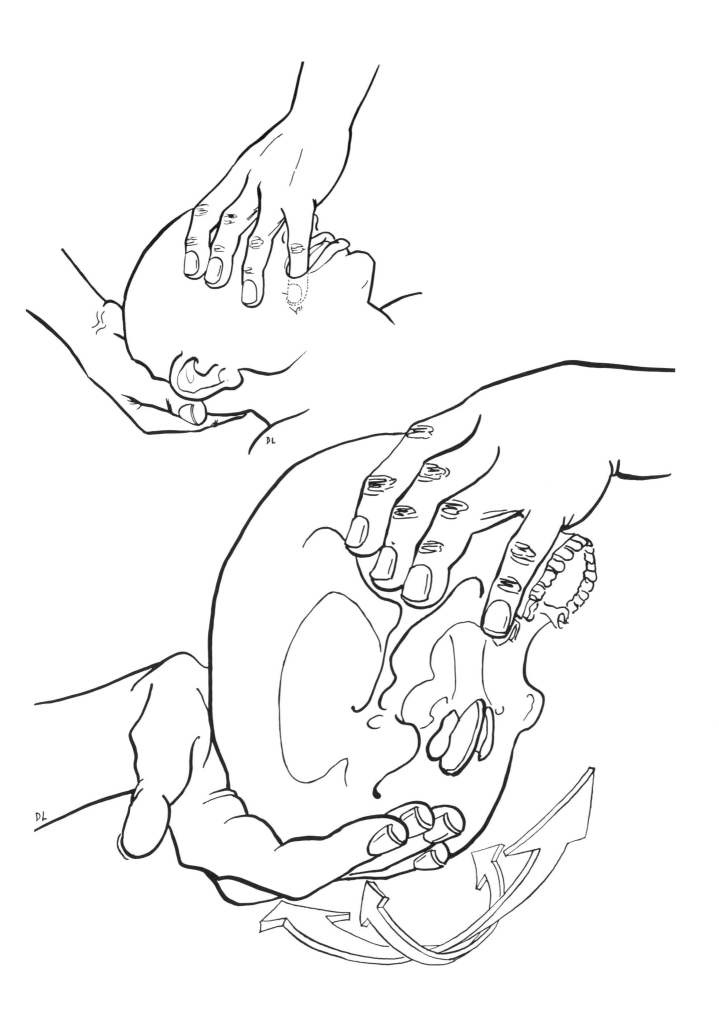

# III  Temporal Techniques

# TEMPORAL BONE MOBILIZATION

### Objective

To correct a temporal bone that is entirely and abnormally fixed or hypomobile within the general motion of the cranium, thus permitting sutural releases and subsequent application of specific treatments.

### Position of the patient

Supine, comfortable and relaxed.

### Position of the practitioner

Seated at the patient's head, forearms resting on the treatment table which has been adjusted to a convenient height.

### Points of contact

With forearm firmly supported by the table, the practitioner follows the temporal into its strain pattern (or lesion) by holding the mastoid process between ring and little fingers, with the middle finger in the external auditory canal and the index finger on the zygomatic process of the temporal.

With the other hand, the practitioner successively acts upon the occiput (nestling the squama transversely in the palm), the parietal (thumb along the temporoparietal suture) and the sphenoid (thumb on the external surface of the greater wing).

### Movement (lesion on the right)

The right hand follows the right temporal to its position of balanced tension. The left hand successively fixes each of the following in position at their maximum physiological amplitude:
- the occiput, by following both flexion (expansion phase) and extension (relaxation phase) to the point of ease;
- the parietal, by releasing the external surface of the parietal (expansion phase) with the thumb;
- the sphenoid, either above the pivot (expansion phase) with the left thumb, or beneath the pivot (relaxation phase) by shifting the external surface of the greater wing anteriorly to the point of ease.

Each position is held until a release is perceived. After all the releases have been obtained, the head is checked carefully for symmetrical motion of the temporals. If this motion is not symmetrical, the appropriate technique described in this chapter is utilized.

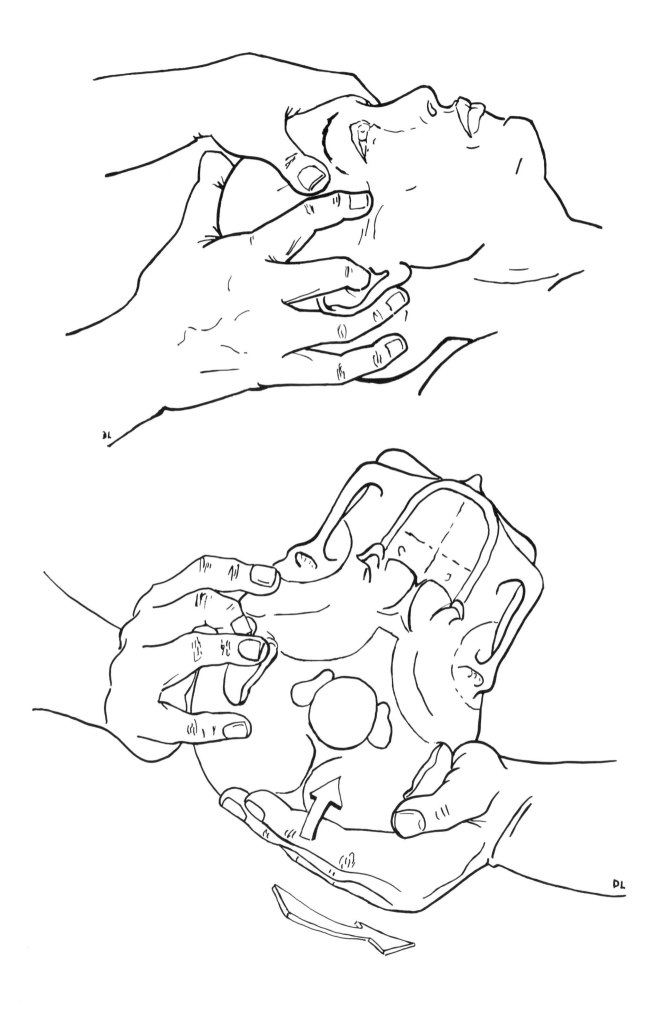

# UNILATERAL EXTERNAL ROTATION

### Objective

To directly reduce a unilateral temporal lesion of internal rotation, or indirectly reduce a unilateral temporal lesion of external rotation.

### Position of the patient

Supine, comfortable and relaxed.

### Position of the practitioner

Seated at the patient's head, forearms resting on the treatment table which has been adjusted to a convenient height.

### Points of contact

The practitioner's hand, on the side of the lesion, controls the temporal as follows:
— the thumb and index finger hold the zygomatic process of the temporal, with the thumb on top and the index finger underneath;
— the ring and the little finger secure the mastoid process, with the ring finger placed anteriorly and the little finger posteriorly.

The occipital squama is cupped in the concavity of the palm of the other hand, placed transversely to the bone.

### Movement (applied to the right)

During the expansion phase, the practitioner's left hand brings about a flexion of the occiput. This is accompanied by a sutural opening on the right caused by a very slight rotation of the occiput toward the left, around its vertical axis.

In synchronization, the practitioner draws the right temporal into external rotation: the thumb and index finger move the zygomatic process caudad and laterally, while the little and middle fingers draw the mastoid process posteriorly and medially.

At the same time, the practitioner asks the patient to turn his or her head slightly and gently to the opposite side (toward the left, in this example). Opposition to that rotation is exerted by the practitioner's occipital hand.

### Comment

This technique must be executed firmly; lesions which require it are commonly caused by trauma.

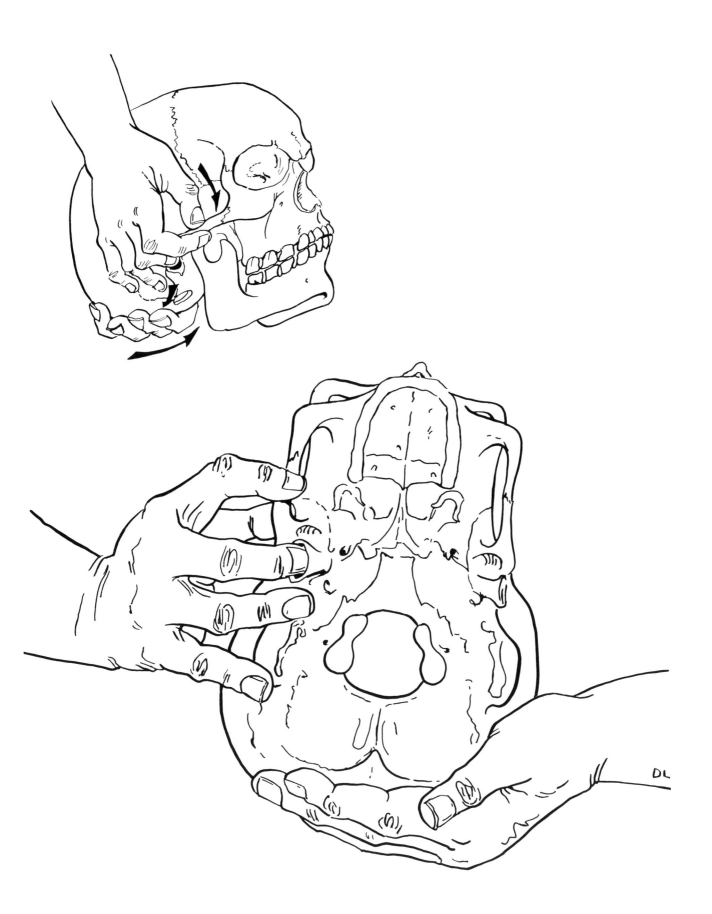

# UNILATERAL INTERNAL ROTATION

### Objective

To directly reduce a unilateral temporal lesion of external rotation, or indirectly reduce a unilateral temporal lesion of internal rotation.

### Position of the patient

Supine, comfortable and relaxed.

### Position of the practitioner

Seated at the patient's head, forearms resting on the treatment table which has been adjusted to a convenient height.

### Points of contact

The practitioner's hand, on the side of the lesion, controls the temporal as follows:
— the thumb and index finger hold the zygomatic process of the temporal, with the thumb above and index finger underneath;
— the ring and little fingers secure the mastoid process, with the ring finger placed anteriorly and the little finger posteriorly.

The occipital squama is cupped in the concavity of the palm of the other hand, positioned transversely to the bone.

### Movement (technique applied to the right)

During the relaxation phase, the practitioner's left hand draws the occiput in extension. This is accompanied by a sutural closing on the right, caused by a very slight rotation of the occiput to the right, around its vertical axis.

In synchronization, the practitioner draws the right temporal into internal rotation: thumb and index finger raise the zygomatic process cephalad and medially, while the little and ring fingers draw the mastoid process anteriorly and laterally. This latter action is reinforced by a posterior and medial pressure of the right thenar eminence on the mastoid portion.

At the same time, the practitioner asks the patient to turn his or her head slightly and gently to the right. Opposition to the rotation is exerted by the practitioner's occipital hand.

### Comment

This technique must be executed firmly; lesions which require it are commonly caused by trauma.

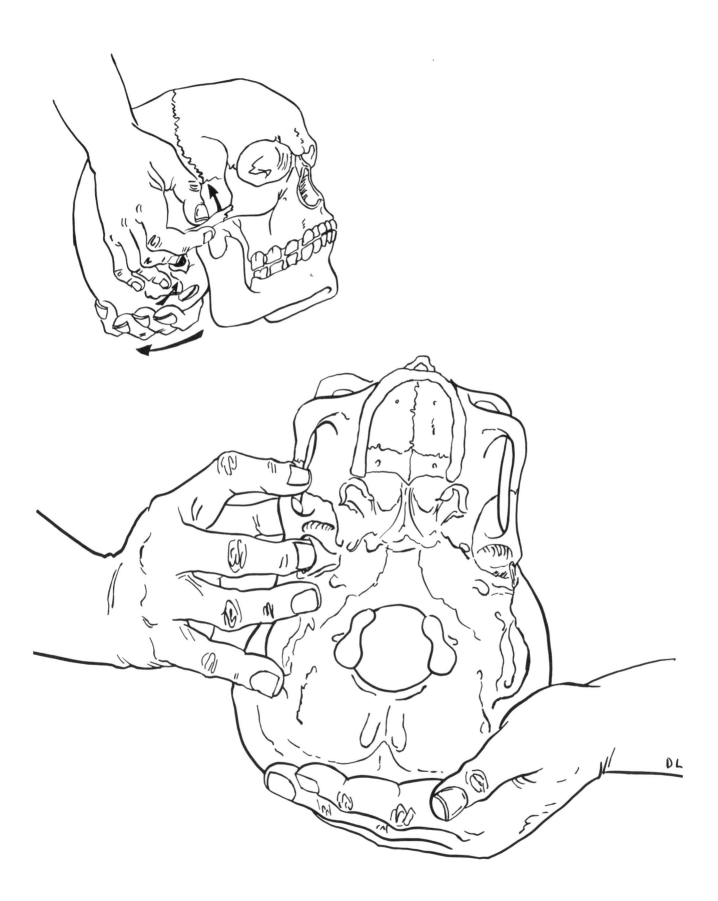

# EUSTACHIAN TUBE TWIST

## Objective

To restore proper functional position to the eustachian tube for good oxygenation as well as drainage of secretions. This requires a normal length of the fibrocartilaginous part, a correct angle with the nasopharynx, and, above all, a patent opening of the isthmus.

This technique acts as a countertwist to the very mild natural twist of the eustachian tube.

## Position of the patient

Supine, comfortable and relaxed.

## Position of the practitioner

Seated at the patient's head, forearms resting on the treatment table which has been adjusted to a convenient height.

## Points of contact

Hands joined, with fingers interlaced under the occiput, the practitioner places his or her thumbs along the mastoid processes.

## Movement (bilateral manipulation)

1st phase: the practitioner exerts a continuous pressure on the mastoid processes caudally and medially (external rotation of the temporals), at the same time lengthening the temporals posteriorly.

2nd phase: the practitioner holds this position while the patient inhales slowly; at the same time the practitioner lays one shoulder against the patient's glabella and exerts a gentle pressure posteriorly.

3rd phase: during the patient's exhalation, the practitioner releases the pressure on the glabella.

4th phase: the 2nd and 3rd phases are repeated until a general relaxation of the tissues is perceived.

## Comment

At the conclusion of this technique, it is necessary to restore the normal relations of the temporals.

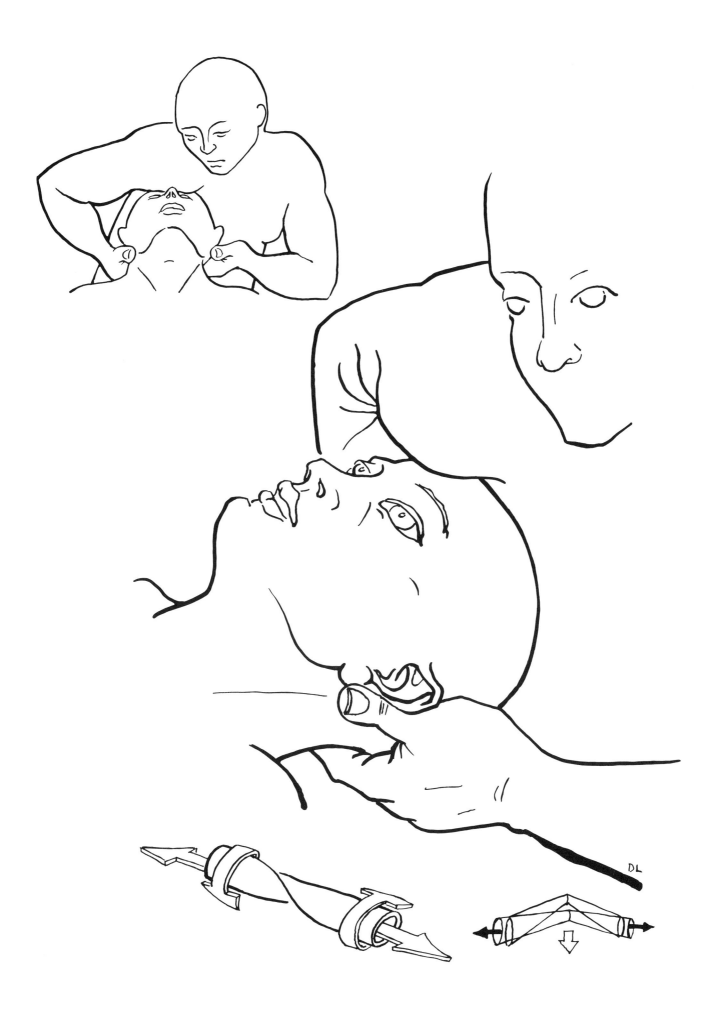

# PETROBASILAR TECHNIQUE

## Objective

To restore the articular harmony of the bones composing the groove of the petrosal portion, in which the occipital groove moves like a hinge.

## Position of the patient

Supine, comfortable and relaxed.

## Position of the practitioner

Seated at the patient's head, forearms resting on the treatment table which has been adjusted to a convenient height.

## Points of contact

One hand controls the temporal in the following manner:
— mastoid process between the little finger posteriorly and the ring finger anteriorly;
— middle finger in the external auditory canal;
— index finger on the zygomatic process of the temporal.
The other hand transversely cradles the occipital squama in the concavity of the palm.

## Movement (lesion on the right)

The hand on the occiput draws it into extension and holds it in position.

During the expansion phase of the cranial mechanism, the right hand brings the right temporal into external rotation: the zygomatic process is directed caudally and laterally, while the mastoid process is directed posteriorly and medially.

This position is held until a release is perceived.

## Comments

This technique, which must be applied after any specific manipulation of the temporal petrosal portion, must be followed by a physiological normalization of the general motion of the cranium.

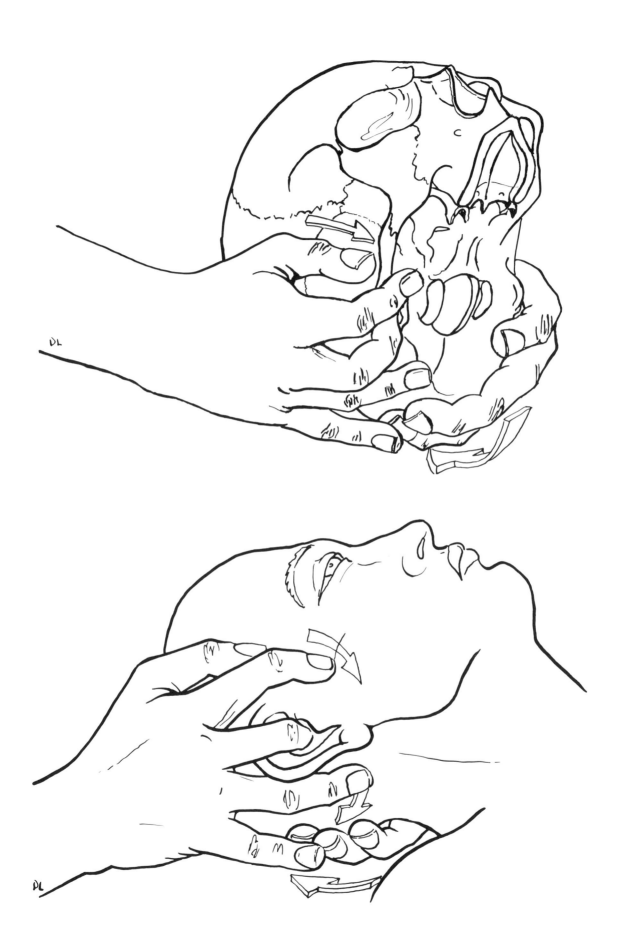

# PETROJUGULAR TECHNIQUE

### Objectives

- To restore the physiological motion between the jugular process of the occiput and the jugular surface of the temporal.
- To stimulate a pumping action at the origin of the jugular vein for drainage.

### Position of the patient

Supine, comfortable and relaxed.

### Position of the practitioner

Seated at the patient's head, forearms resting on the treatment table which has been adjusted to a convenient height.

### Points of contact

One hand, the forearm of which is perpendicular to the longitudinal axis of the cranium, controls the temporal as follows:
- —the thumb on the zygomatic process, the index finger underneath;
- —the tip of the middle finger in the external auditory canal;
- —the ring finger in the anterior portion of the digastric groove;
- —the little finger behind the mastoid process.

The other hand transversely cradles the occipital squama in the hollow of the palm.

### Movement (lesion on the right)

At the same time that the practitioner externally rotates the temporal, he or she raises and draws it apart from the occiput: the thumb and index clamp emphasizes the lateral aspect of its movement; the bone is drawn laterally along the axis of the practitioner's forearm; and, simultaneously, the ring finger draws aside the mastoid process.

The left hand carries along the occiput in flexion, anteriorly and caudally, during the expansion phase of the cranial mechanism.

This technique stimulates venous drainage when applied rhythmically during successive expansion phases of the cranial mechanism, alternating with passivity during the relaxation phases.

92

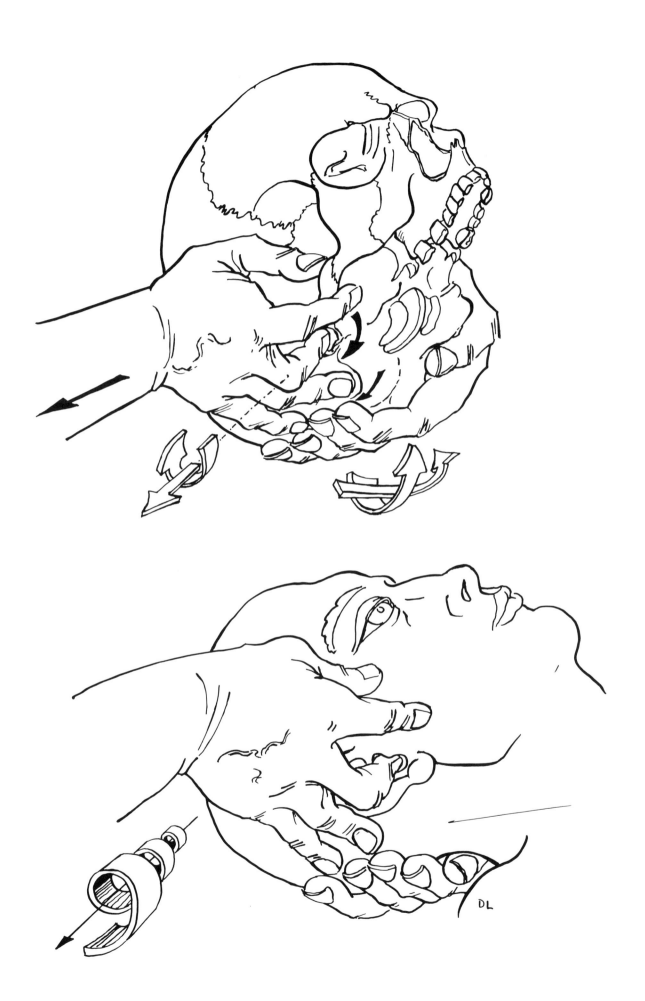

# PARIETOMASTOID TECHNIQUE

### Objective

To restore the parietomastoid functional relationship.

### Position of the patient

Supine, comfortable and relaxed, with a slight rotation of the head toward the side opposite the lesion.

### Position of the practitioner

Seated at the patient's head on the side of the lesion, with the treatment table adjusted to a convenient height.

### Points of contact

One thumb is placed on the mastoid process (on the corresponding side of the head), with the thenar eminence near the affected suture.

The thumb of the other hand is placed on the posteroinferior angle of the parietal, with the distal phalanx pointing toward the thenar eminence of the other thumb. The remainder of the hand is spread out on the parietals.

### Movement (lesion on the right)

During the expansion phase of the cranial mechanism, the right thumb presses slightly on the mastoid process, while rolling laterally (along its longitudinal axis) and sliding posteriorly.

At the same time, the left thumb rolls medially (around its longitudinal axis) while sliding anteriorly and slightly cephalad. This is reinforced by a very light traction along the axis of the nail and the base of the thumb, toward the thenar eminence. This position is held until a release is perceived.

### Comment

When this technique is ineffective, that on page 96 is utilized.

94

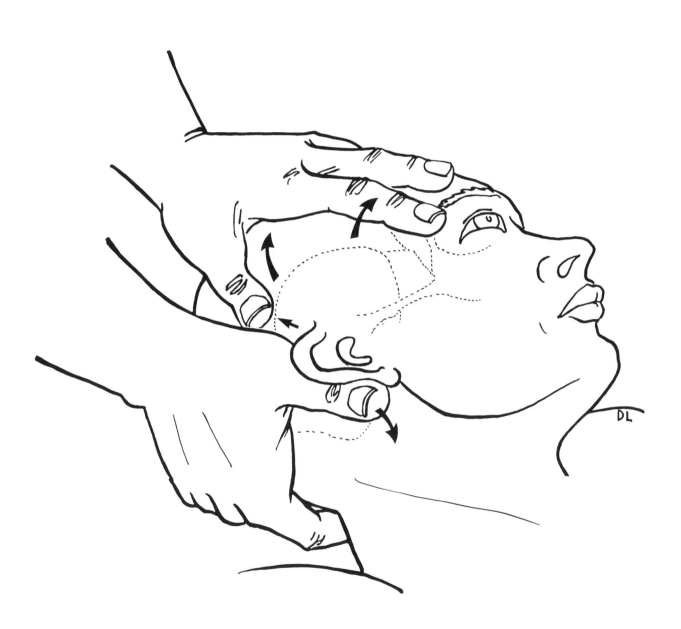

# PARIETOMASTOID PIVOT

### Objective

To restore free functional mobility in the parietomastoid area when there is internal rotation of the temporal bone together with a depression of the area immediately posterior to the auricle.

### Position of the patient

Supine, comfortable and relaxed.

### Position of the practitioner

Seated at the patient's head on the side of the lesion, the treatment table adjusted to a convenient height.

### Points of contact

The hand on the lesion side cradles the posterior lateral aspect of the cranium in its palm, while the thumb controls the mastoid process along the anterior border.

The other hand cups the parietal bones in the palm, thumb on the posteroinferior angle on the side of the lesion.

### Movement (lesion on the right)

The movement consists of two successive, perfectly coordinated phases.

1st phase:  during the relaxation phase of the cranial mechanism, the hand on the temporal bone follows it into the lesion pattern. The temporal is drawn into internal rotation, while the mastoid process moves cephalad and the squama is maintained medially.

The other hand exaggerates the flattened position of the parietal bone by pressing the thumb caudally and medially on the posteroinferior angle.

2nd phase:  the lesion is reduced during the expansion phase of the cranial mechanism. The left hand thumb draws the posteroinferior angle of the right parietal anteriorly and cephalad, with the other fingers helping this external rotation. At the same time, the right hand encourages external rotation of the right temporal (mastoid process posterior and caudal).

At the same time, the patient is required to sidebend his or her head slightly to the left. This position is held until a release is perceived.

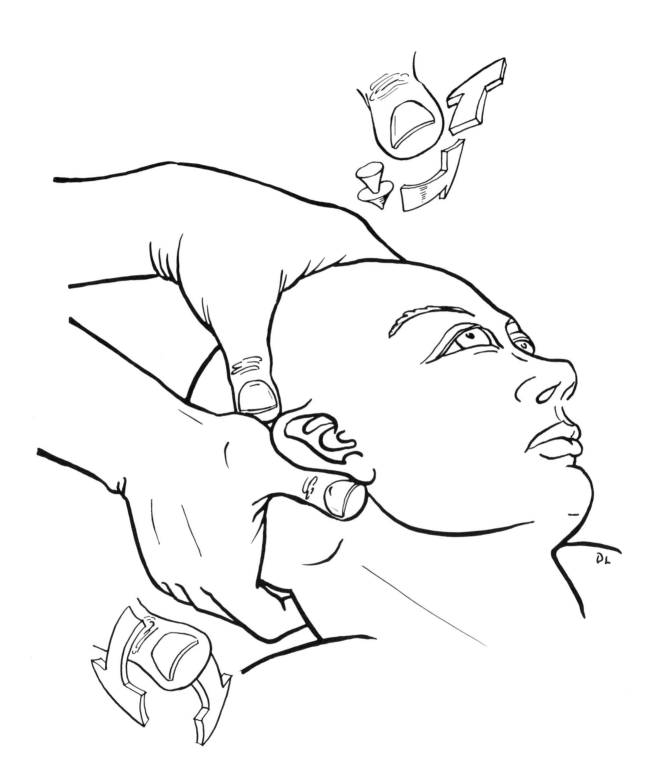

# RELEASE OF THE TEMPOROPARIETAL SUTURE

### Objective

To restore normal mobility to the temporoparietal suture and thereby restore functional harmony to the cranial mechanism, particularly allowing for sufficient lateral expansion during the phases of cranial motion.

### Position of the patient

Supine, comfortable and relaxed, head turned slightly to the side opposite the lesion.

### Position of the practitioner

Seated at the patient's head on the side of the lesion, with the treatment table adjusted to a convenient height.

### Points of contact

The thumbs are parallel and separated by the temporoparietal suture. The thumb of the cephalic hand is on the parietal bone, and the thumb of the caudal hand on the temporal squama on either side of a restricted area. The latter also touches the mastoid portion on the lesion side, with the palmar surface of the thumb at the base of the first phalanx of the index finger.

### Movement (manipulation on the right side)

1st phase:  during the relaxation phase of the cranial mechanism, the left thumb on the parietal (external bevel) releases that bone by exerting pressure medially.

2nd phase:  when the expansion phase is starting, this same thumb draws its point of contact cephalad and anteriorly, while the other hand encourages external rotation of the temporal. The practitioner draws the mastoid portion caudally and posteriorly by pressure at the base of the first phalanx of the index finger. At the same time, the thumb of this hand tries to increase the gap between itself and the other thumb. This position is held until a release is perceived.

### Comments

Severe restrictions may require maintaining the external rotation of the temporal for some time, or a combination of this technique and the temporal bone mobilization described on page 82 above.

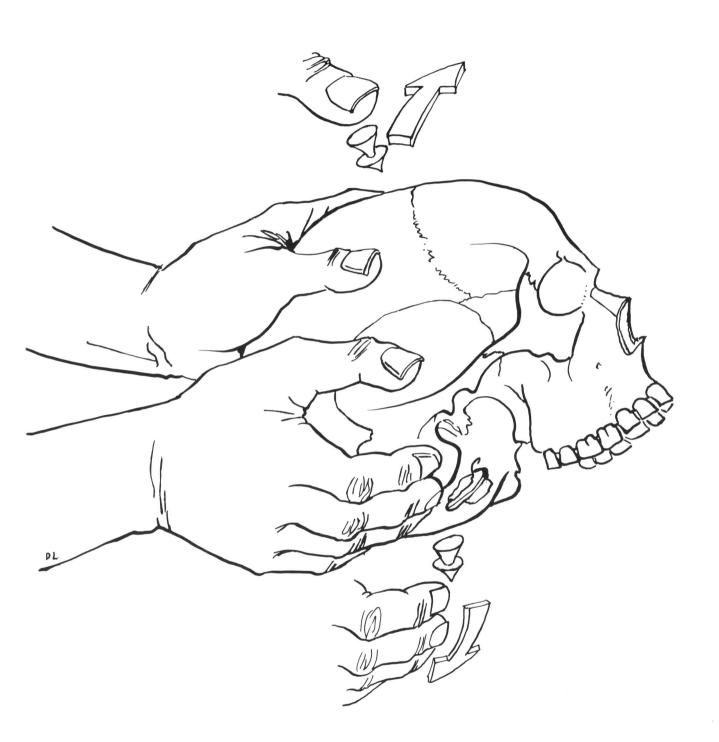

DL

# SPHENOSQUAMOUS PIVOT

## SUPERIOR BEVEL

### Objective

To release the superior bevel (i.e., the external surface on the greater wing of the sphenoid to the internal surface on the temporal) of the sphenosquamous pivot.

### Position of the patient

Supine, comfortable and relaxed.

### Position of the practitioner

Seated at the patient's head on the side of the lesion, at the corner of the treatment table. The forearm on the side of the lesion rests on the table, which has been adjusted to a convenient height.

### Points of contact

The supine hand on the side of the lesion envelops the upper cervical spine. The thumb is placed along the mastoid process, the thenar eminence touching the mastoid portion of the temporal.

The palm of the other hand cups the frontal bone. The thumb is placed on the greater wing of the sphenoid, on the side of the lesion. The other fingers point obliquely toward the opposite external orbital process.

### Movement (manipulation on the right side)

Each of the following phases must be performed in smooth and overlapping succession, without abruptness, one movement beginning as another is phased out.

1st phase: during the expansion phase, by a gentle and constant pressure, the practitioner draws the temporal bone in external rotation.

2nd phase: during the relaxation phase, the left hand releases the greater wing by drawing it in a slightly posterior and primarily medial direction. This action can be reinforced if the patient rotates his head slightly toward the right.

3rd phase: during the expansion phase, the practitioner exerts a gentle and constant pressure on the greater wing. The pressure is exerted in successively straight anterior (along the anteroposterior axis), anterior (around the transverse axis), and medial (around the vertical axis) directions. At the same time, the patient must turn his head somewhat to the left.

This technique should be applied several times until a release is perceived, the practitioner taking care to respect the different phases of the cranial mechanism.

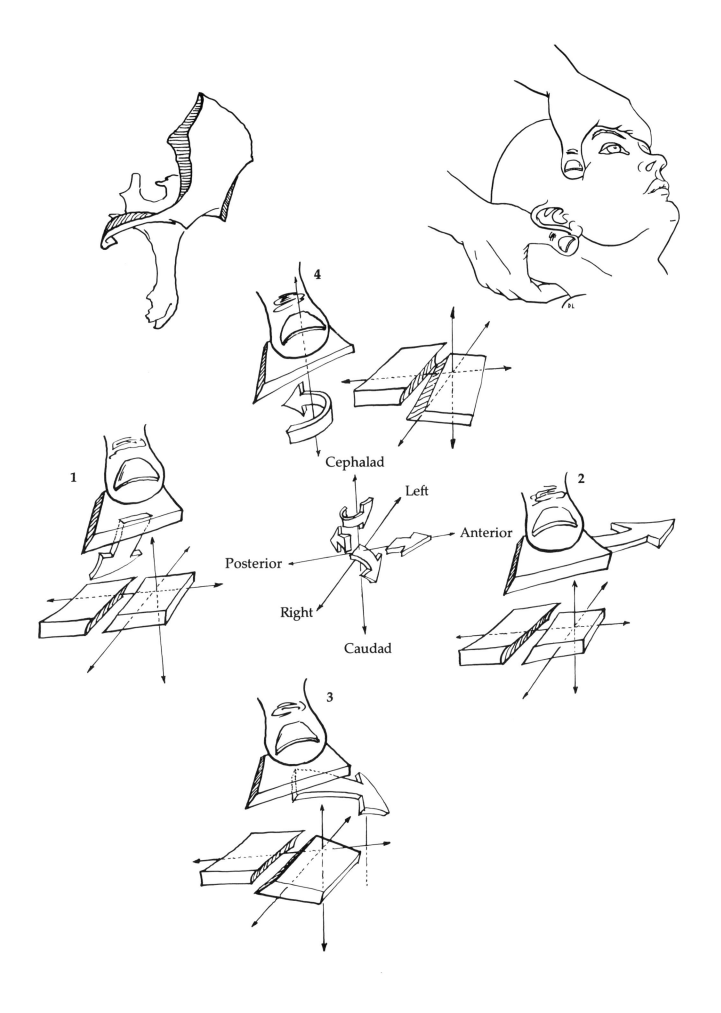

**4**

Cephalad

Left

Anterior

Posterior

Right

Caudad

**1**

**2**

**3**

# SPHENOSQUAMOUS PIVOT

## INFERIOR BEVEL

**Objective**

To release the inferior bevel (internal surface on the greater wing of the sphenoid to the external surface on the temporal) of the sphenosquamous pivot.

**Position of the patient**

Supine, comfortable and relaxed.

**Position of the practitioner**

Seated at the patient's head, on the side of the lesion, near the corner of the treatment table. The forearm on the side of the lesion rests on the treatment table, which has been adjusted to a convenient height.

**Points of contact**

The supine hand on the side of the lesion envelops the upper cervical spine. The thumb is placed along the mastoid process, the thenar eminence touching the mastoid portion of the temporal.

The palm of the other hand cups the frontal bone. The thumb is placed on the greater wing of the sphenoid on the side of the lesion. The other fingers point obliquely toward the opposite external orbital process.

**Movement** (technique applied on the right)

Like the previous technique, there must be a smooth and overlapping succession of the consecutive phases.

1st phase:   during the expansion phase of cranial motion, the practitioner presses on the mastoid process gently and with a constant force, to initiate an external rotation of the temporal.

2nd phase:   during the relaxation phase, the left hand draws the greater wing in a caudal and slightly lateral direction, to release the inferior bevel. This action is reinforced by a slight rotation of the patient's head to the opposite side.

3rd phase:   during the expansion phase, the practitioner moves the greater wing in a successively anterior (transverse axis), cephalad (anteroposterior axis) and medial (vertical axis) direction, while the patient turns his or her head to the left.

This technique must be applied several times until a release is perceived, the practitioner taking care to respect the different phases of the cranial mechanism.

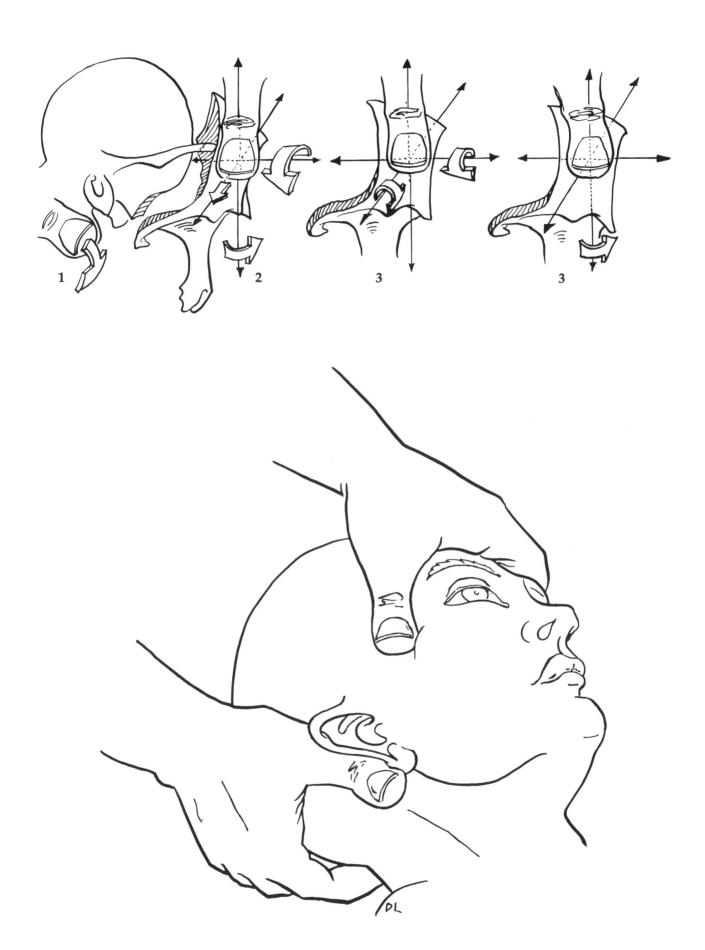

# DECOMPRESSION OF THE SPHENOSQUAMOUS PIVOT

## FIRST TECHNIQUE

### Objective

To release a compression affecting the whole sphenosquamous pivot.

### Position of the patient

Supine, comfortable and relaxed.

### Position of the practitioner

Seated at the patient's head, on the side of the lesion, near the corner of the treatment table. The forearm on the lesion side rests on the table, which has been adjusted to a convenient height.

### Points of contact

The practitioner's supine hand on the side of the lesion envelops the upper cervical spine. The thumb is placed along the mastoid process, the thenar eminence touching the mastoid portion of the temporal.

The palm of the other hand cups the frontal bone. The thumb is placed on the greater wing of the sphenoid, on the side of the lesion. The other fingers point obliquely toward the opposite external orbital process.

### Movement (technique applied on the right)

1st phase: during the expansion phase, the practitioner presses with gentle and constant force on the right mastoid process, so as to draw the right temporal into external rotation.

2nd phase: during the relaxation phase, the left hand releases the external bevel of the greater wing by drawing it in a medial and slightly posterior direction, and releases the internal bevel (under the pivot point) by bringing it caudad (around the anteroposterior axis).

3rd phase: during the expansion phase, the left hand pulls the sphenoid anteriorly, thus increasing the separation from the temporal. This action of the left hand can be reinforced by the rotation of the patient's head to the left (around a vertical axis) at the end of the movement.

This position is held until a release and a new balance point is perceived.

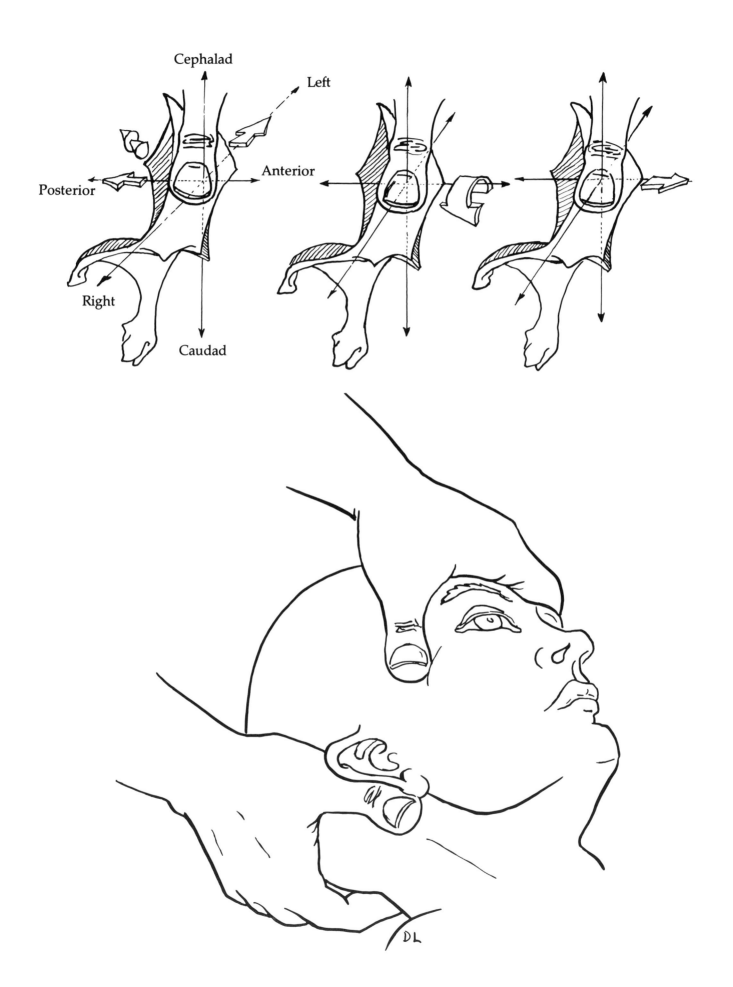

Cephalad

Left

Anterior

Posterior

Right

Caudad

# DECOMPRESSION OF THE SPHENOSQUAMOUS PIVOT

## SECOND TECHNIQUE

**Objective**

To release a compression affecting the whole sphenosquamous pivot.

**Position of the patient**

Supine, comfortable and relaxed.

**Position of the practitioner**

Seated at the patient's head, on the side of the lesion. The corresponding forearm rests on the treatment table, which has been adjusted to a convenient height.

**Points of contact**

The practitioner's hand, on the side of the patient's lesion, touches the temporal as follows:
— index finger in the external auditory canal;
— middle finger (reinforced posteriorly by the ring finger) in the digastric groove.

The other hand controls the anterior part of the cranium on the side of the lesion with the following contact points:
— little finger, intrabuccal, on the external surface of the pterygoid process;
— middle finger on the greater wing of the sphenoid;
— index finger on the adjacent frontal eminence.

**Movement** (technique applied on the right)

1st phase:   during the expansion phase, the practitioner draws the temporal into external rotation.

2nd phase:   during the relaxation phase, the middle finger of the left hand moves the greater wing in a caudal and primarily medial direction, thus releasing both bevels of the sphenosquamous pivot.

3rd phase:   during the expansion phase, the middle finger then draws the greater wing anteriorly, while the little finger controls the flexion of the sphenoid at the pterygoid process. This movement is aided by the support of the index finger on the frontal eminence, allowing the rotation of the sphenoid around the vertical axis.

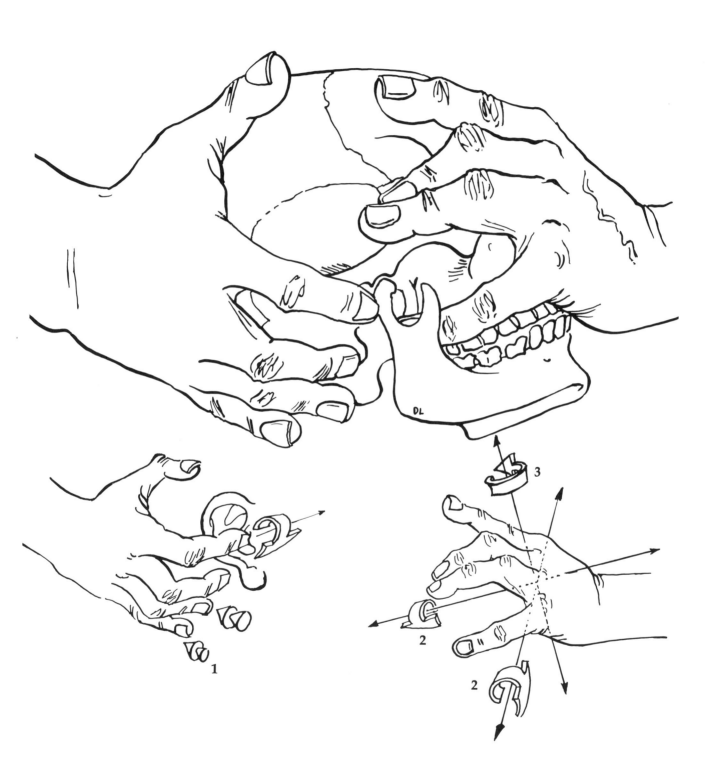

1

2

2

3

DL

# SPHENOPETROSAL REPOSITIONING

**Objective**

To restore the functional and anatomical connections of the elements of the sphenopetrosal articulation in all spatial planes.

**Position of the patient**

Supine, comfortable and relaxed.

**Position of the practitioner**

Seated at the patient's head, on the side opposite the lesion. The corresponding forearm rests on the treatment table, which has been adjusted to a convenient height.

**Points of contact**

The practitioner's supine hand, on the side opposite the patient's lesion, cups the upper cervical spine. The thumb is placed along the mastoid process, with the thenar eminence contacting the mastoid portion of the temporal on the side of the lesion.

The other hand, enveloping the frontal bone, controls the repositioning of the sphenoid. The thumb is on the greater wing, on the side opposite the lesion. The index finger (and/or middle finger) is on the other greater wing, on the side of the lesion. The little finger is positioned on the external surface of the pterygoid process.

**Movement** (technique applied to the right)

The practitioner's right hand draws the corresponding temporal bone in external rotation. The left hand controls the sphenoid, repositioning it around its transverse, anteroposterior and vertical axes. This point of balanced tension is held until a release is perceived.

In an acceptable variation, the hand on the temporal (in this example, the right one) can control it in a manner described on page 106.

**Comments**

It is essential that adequate testing be done and that this repositioning technique be performed with strict respect for the cranial mechanism, because of the relatively great mobility of this articulation and the importance of the sphenopetrosal ligament.

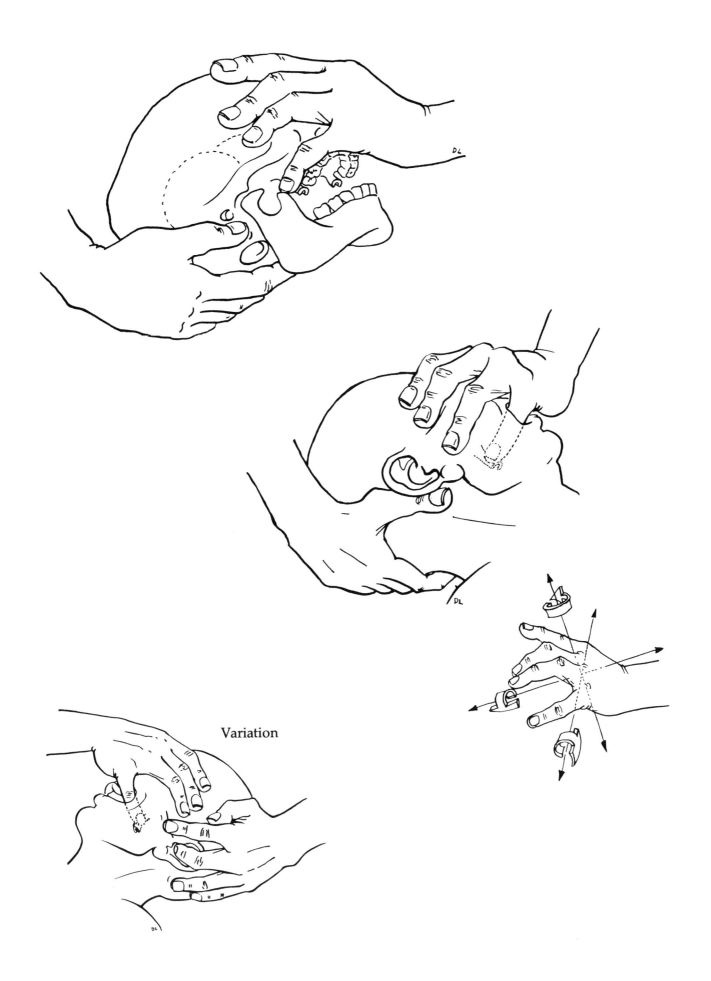

Variation

# TEMPOROZYGOMATIC TECHNIQUE

## Objective

To free the temporozygomatic articulation in the three spatial planes.

## Position of the patient

Supine, comfortable and relaxed.

## Position of the practitioner

Seated at the patient's head on the side opposite the lesion. The caudal forearm is over the patient's chest, without touching it. The treatment table has been adjusted to a convenient height.

## Points of contact

The cephalic hand mobilizes the temporal bone, as follows:
— the ring finger (in front) and the little finger (behind) frame the mastoid process;
— the middle finger is in the external auditory canal;
— the thumb (above) and the index finger (beneath) control the zygomatic process of the temporal.

The caudal hand holds the zygoma gently between the thumb externally and the intra-buccal index finger.

## Movement

The two hands set the temporozygomatic articulation in motion by opposing twists along the axis of the temporozygomatic articulation. When the release has been perceived, the zygoma is taken to the point of balanced tension along the posteroanterior and transverse axes. Because of the slight amount of free motion at the articulation, this very gentle maneuver must be performed with great care.

## Comment

Because the zygomatic lever is short, the practitioner must avoid setting this bone in motion only in relation to the temporal bone, which is more or less immobilized in external rotation. This would risk altering the relationship between the zygoma and the maxilla when the general motion of the cranium is resumed.

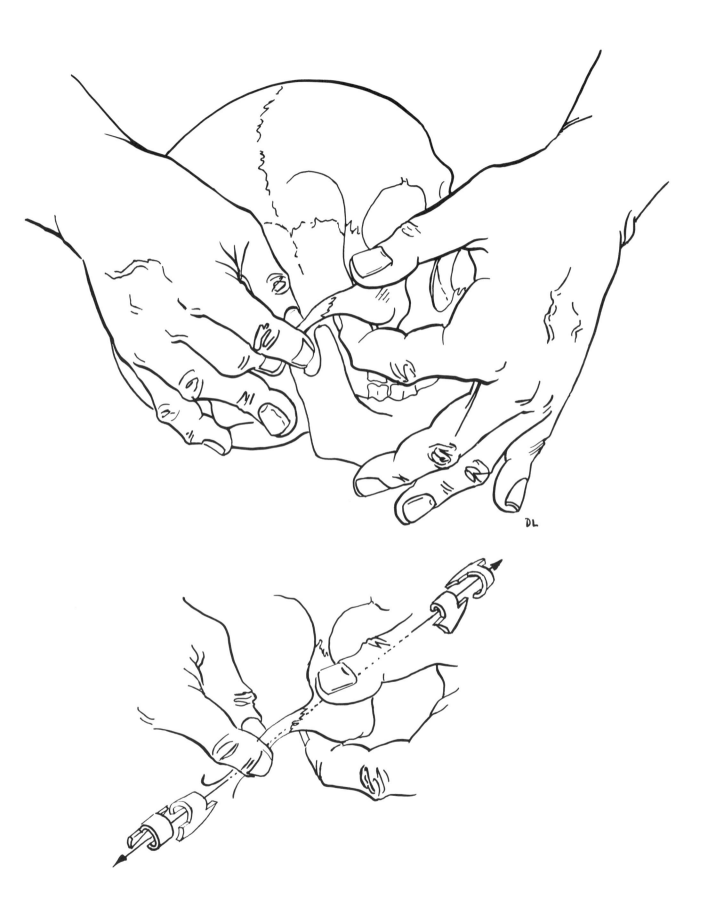

# IV  Frontal Techniques

# FRONTAL SPREAD

**Objectives**

- To allow the frontal bone to perform its physiological motion during the expansion phase of the cranial mechanism.
- To widen the posterior ethmoidal notch of the frontal bone, which is often a very important site of restriction.

**Position of the patient**

Supine, comfortable and relaxed.

**Position of the practitioner**

Seated at the patient's head, the treatment table adjusted to a convenient height.

**Points of contact**

The practitioner's hands control each frontal as follows:
—thumbs are either crossed on the metopic suture or are parallel to it, acting as the base point for the muscular action of this technique;
—the radial side of the index finger is tucked behind the external orbital process.

**Movement**

During the expansion phase of the cranial mechanism, the practitioner synchronizes his or her actions at the two contact points by depressing the glabella posterosuperiorly with the thumbs, and drawing the external orbital processes anteriorly with the index fingers. The external rotation of the frontal bone is facilitated when the index fingers are slightly supinated.

**Comment**

This technique permits a very wide range of variations, acting locally on any part of the frontal bone.

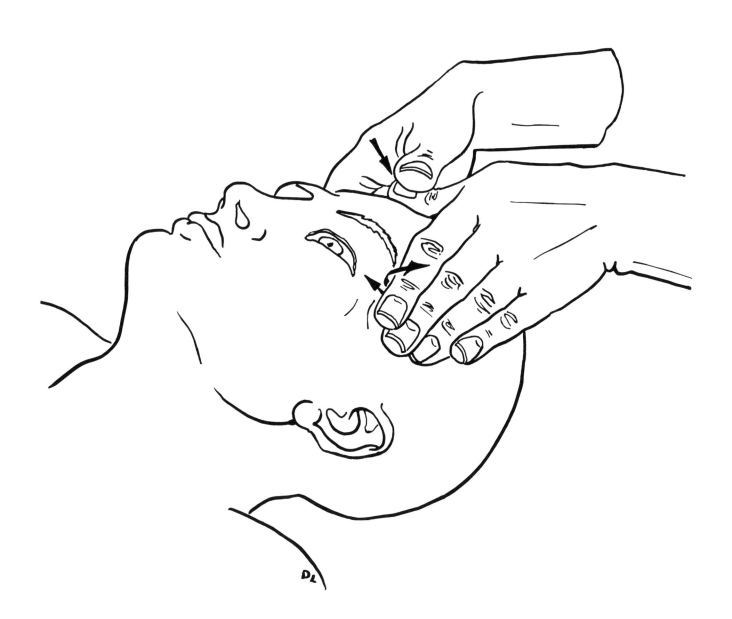

# FRONTAL LIFT

## INTERNAL ROTATION

### Objectives

- To allow the frontal bone to perform its normal physiological motion during the relaxation phase of the cranial mechanism.
- To free the inferior aspects of the coronal suture.

### Position of the patient

Supine, comfortable and relaxed.

### Position of the practitioner

Seated at the patient's head, body bent slightly forward, with the table adjusted to a convenient height.

### Points of contact

The practitioner interlaces his or her fingers above the metopic suture. The hypothenar eminences are then placed on the corresponding lateral angles of the frontal bone, with the heel of the hand in front of the coronal suture.

### Movement

During the relaxation phase of the cranial mechanism, the practitioner's interlaced fingers exert a gentle, even and constant pressure against each other. This results in medial pressure against the frontal eminences via the hypothenar eminences. The practitioner then raises the frontal anteriorly either unilaterally or bilaterally, as appropriate to the diagnosis.

In the case of a unilateral lesion, the practitioner may add a rotation around the vertical axis of the frontal toward the opposite side.

### Comment

This technique must occasionally be preceded by the reduction of any lesion at the rough and irregular L-shaped surface between the frontal and the greater wing of the sphenoid.

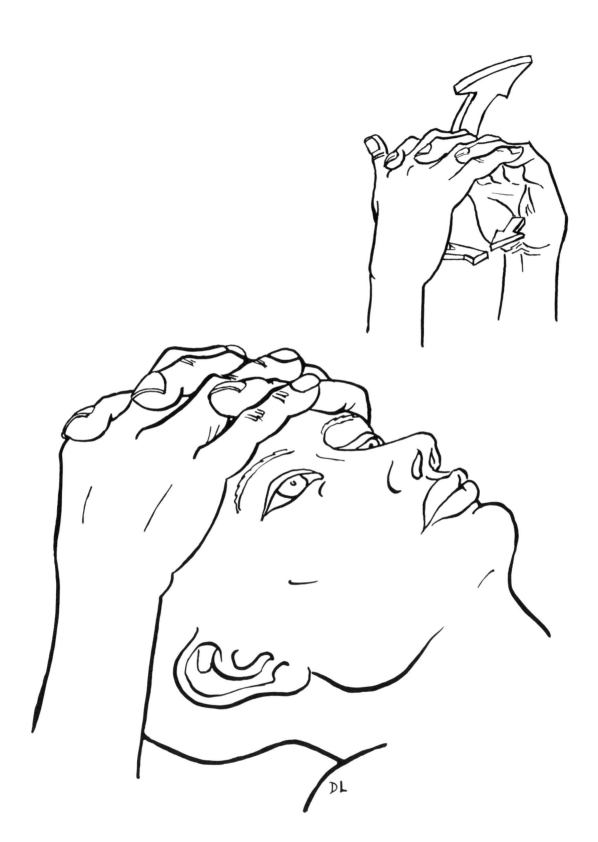

# DECOMPRESSION OF THE FRONTAL BONE

**Objective**

To promote the physiological motions of flexion-extension of the frontal to the maximum amplitude. In order to assure a perfect functional freedom, there is also an element of lifting involved.

**Position of the patient**

Supine, comfortable and relaxed.

**Position of the practitioner**

Seated at the patient's head, body bent slightly forward over the patient's cranium. The treatment table has been adjusted to a convenient height.

**Points of contact**

The practitioner interlaces his or her fingers above the metopic suture. The practitioner then positions the hypothenar eminences on the corresponding lateral angles of the frontal bone, with the heels of the hands in front of the coronal suture.

**Movement**

1st phase: during the relaxation phase of the cranial mechanism, the practitioner's interlaced fingers exert a gentle, even and constant medial pressure via the hypothenar eminences. The practitioner then raises the frontal anteriorly.

2nd phase: during the expansion phase, without releasing the pressure, the practitioner draws the frontal bone into flexion.

3rd phase: during the relaxation phase in this new position, the practitioner continues the medial pressure, raising the frontal cephalad to the limit allowed by the soft tissues.

4th phase: the practitioner repeats the second phase. The cycle continues until a release signals freedom of the frontal bone. A check for the degree of freedom can be made using one of the holds described at the beginning of this book (pages 10 & 12), or with movement tests.

**Comment**

This technique requires a sensitivity to the cranial mechanism if the patient is to feel no discomfort. Sensitivity of this degree is usually found only among moderately experienced practitioners, who must be able to continuously appraise the changing condition of the various tissues.

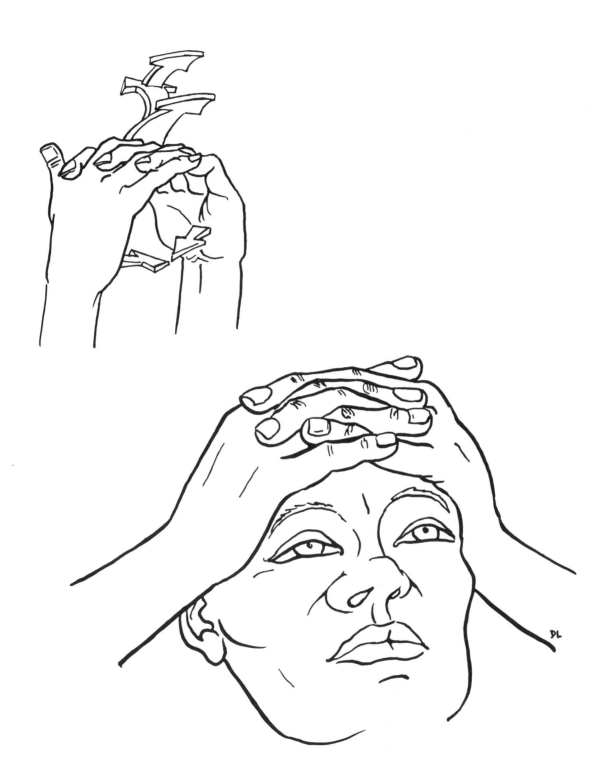

# FRONTOSPHENOIDAL RELEASE: GREATER WING

## "CANT HOOK"

### Objective

To free the frontosphenoidal area at the L-shaped surface of the greater wing of the sphenoid, particularly in cases of unilateral impaction, which occur frequently in this area.

### Position of the patient

Supine, comfortable and relaxed.

### Position of the practitioner

Seated at the patient's head, on the side opposite the lesion, the treatment table adjusted to a convenient height.

### Points of contact

The practitioner stabilizes the sphenoid with the caudal hand by placing the fingers as follows:

— little finger, intrabuccal, on the external surface of the pterygoid process on the side of the lesion;

— index finger on the greater wing of the sphenoid on the side of the lesion;

— thumb on the other greater wing.

The other hand controls the frontal bone as follows:

— thumb above and against the thumb of the caudal hand, providing support during the movement;

— index and middle fingers placed on the side of the lesion under the temporal line of the frontal.

### Movement

While the caudal hand supports the sphenoid (generally in its lesion position), the cephalic hand, basing itself on the thumb, brings about the disimpaction until a release is perceived. This action requires a lifting movement anteriorly around the transverse axis, and toward the non-lesioned side around the anteroposterior axis. In order to increase the technique's efficacy, the cephalic hand may perform slight, oscillating tremor-like movements.

To complete the technique, the practitioner is encouraged to pass from one axis to the other for several cycles of the cranial rhythm to obtain the freedom of the L-shaped surface.

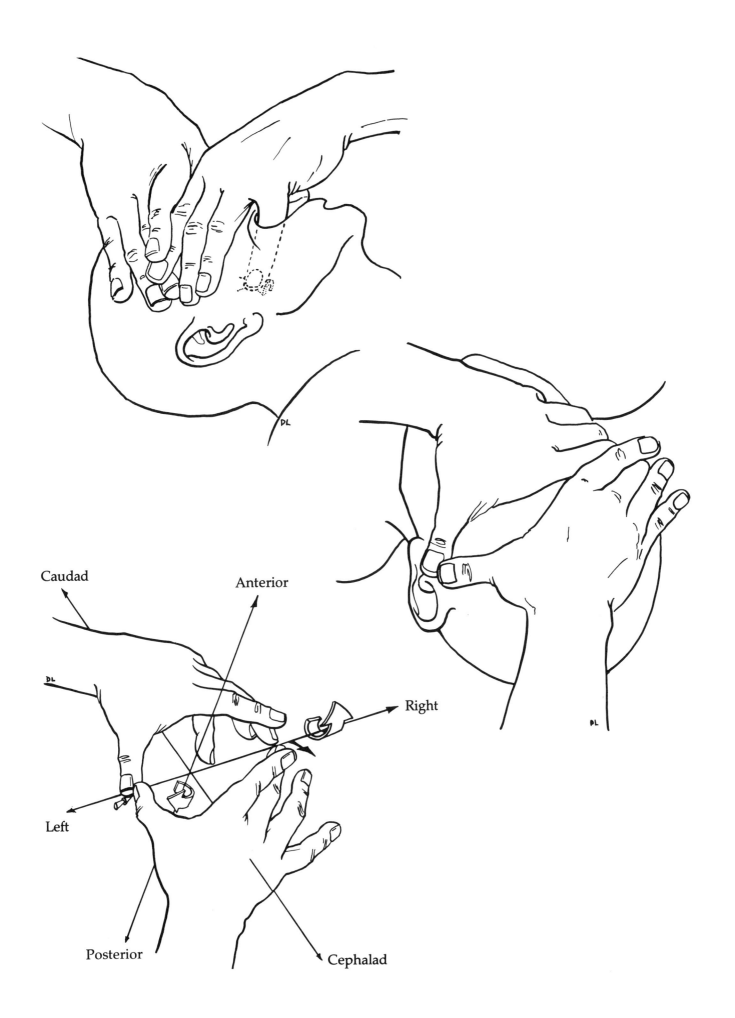

Caudad

Anterior

Right

Left

Posterior

Cephalad

# FRONTOSPHENOIDAL RELEASE: LESSER WING

**Objective**

To free the frontosphenoidal articulation at the lesser wing.

**Position of the patient**

Supine, comfortable and relaxed.

**Position of the practitioner**

Seated at one side of the patient's head, the treatment table adjusted to a convenient height. If the lesion is unilateral, the practitioner sits on the side opposite the lesion.

**Points of contact**

The caudal hand immobilizes the sphenoid in the following manner:
— index and/or middle finger on the external surface of the greater wing;
— thumb, on the practitioner's side, on the opposite greater wing;
— little finger, intrabuccal, on the external surface of the pterygoid process.

The cephalic hand controls the frontal bone in the following manner:
— palm cupping the bone, in front of the coronal suture;
— thumb under the temporal line on the practitioner's side;
— index and middle finger under the same line, but on the opposite side.

**Movement**

The caudal hand immobilizes the sphenoid in its position of balanced tension.

Release of the internal bevel: the cephalic hand accompanies the frontal bone in flexion, then lifts it anteriorly and caudally. The release is increased by small, in-and-out movements along the transverse axis which are begun at the end of flexion.

Release of the external bevel: the cephalic hand performs the same vertical maneuver, but this time toward the vertex. The small, in-and-out movements also accompany this maneuver.

When a unilateral lesion occurs, the movement described above is performed on the side opposite the practitioner, with the thumb of the cephalic hand based firmly on the side opposite the lesion.

In an acceptable variation, the little finger of the caudal hand is placed externally on the maxilla.

**Comment**

The motion of the frontosphenoidal articulation at the lesser wing is very minute, and can be perceived only by experienced practitioners.

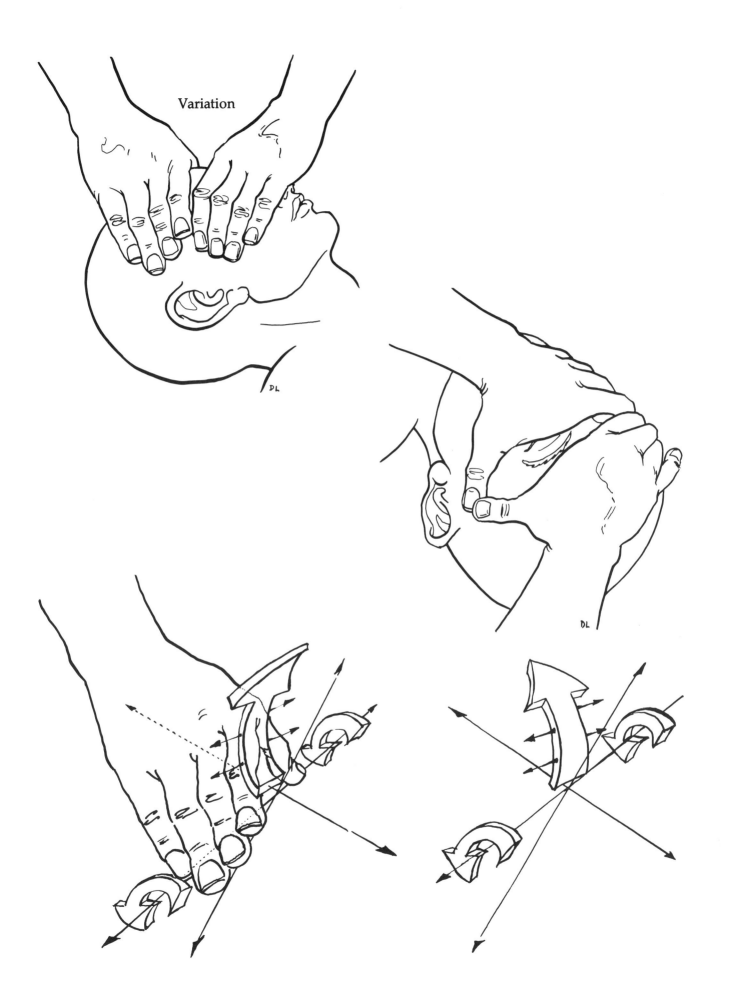

Variation

# FRONTOSPHENOIDAL RELEASE: LESSER WING

## VAULT HOLD

### Objective

To free the frontosphenoidal articulation at the lesser wing. This technique is gentler than the one described on page 122, and is insufficient to bring about, for example, a post-traumatic disengagement.

### Movement

Using the vault hold (page 10), and during the expansion phase of the cranial mechanism, the following movements are performed simultaneously:

— the little fingers stabilize the occiput posteriorly, so as to increase the tension on the tentorium cerebelli (which locks the lesser wings of the sphenoid posteriorly);

— the middle fingers are positioned on the greater wings of the sphenoid and support them caudally;

— the index fingers, placed behind the external orbital process of the frontal, raise the lateral angles of this bone anteriorly.

These movements are sustained until a new balance is reached.

### Comment

The motion of the frontosphenoidal articulation at the lesser wing is very minute and can be perceived only by experienced practitioners. The symmetrical position of the hands in this particular technique enhances the quality and accuracy of the practitioner's perceptions.

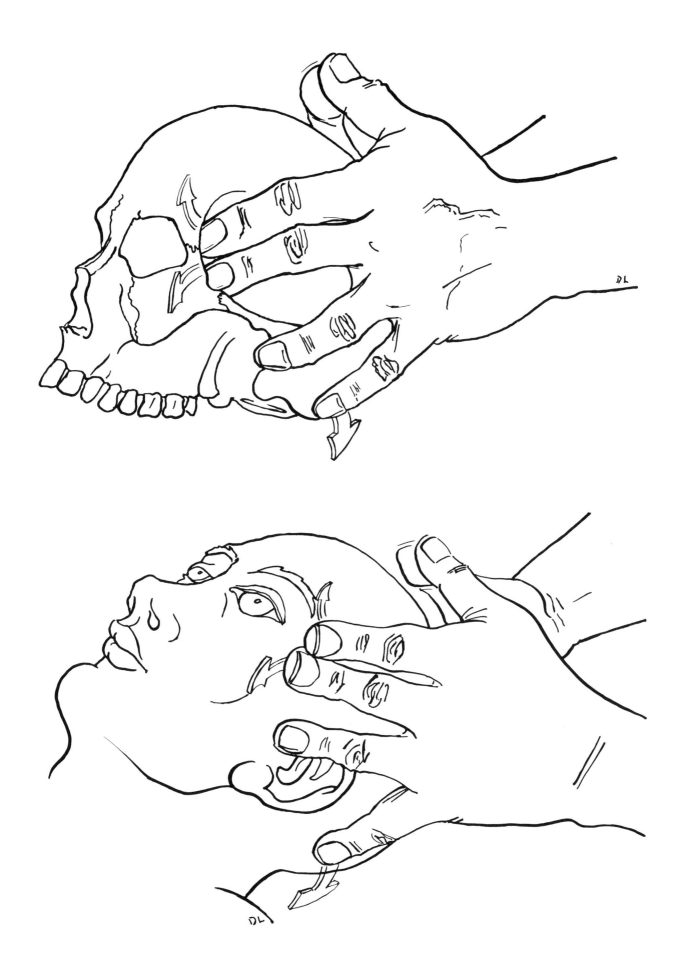

# FRONTOZYGOMATIC TECHNIQUE

### Objective

To free the articulation between the zygomatic process of the frontal bone and the frontal process of the zygoma.

### Position of the patient

Supine, comfortable and relaxed.

### Position of the practitioner

Seated at the patient's head, shifted very slightly to the side of the lesion. The practitioner's forearm on the side of the lesion rests on the treatment table, which has been adjusted to a convenient height.

### Points of contact

The practitioner's hand on the side of the lesion immobilizes the zygoma in external rotation, between the index finger (above) and the middle finger (below).

The other hand controls the frontal as follows:
— palm of the hand cupping the frontal, in front of the coronal suture;
— thumb behind the external orbital process, on the side of the lesion;
— index and/or middle finger behind the external orbital process, on the opposite side.

### Movement

While the hand on the side of the lesion completely immobilizes the zygoma in external rotation, the other hand draws the frontal bone in flexion during the expansion phase of the cranial mechanism. At the end of the movement, the latter hand very slightly exaggerates the anterior displacement of the external orbital process of the frontal, while simultaneously inducing a gentle cephalad rotation around its transverse axis. This is held until a release is perceived.

### Comment

An alternative to this technique would be for the practitioner to position himself or herself on the other side of the patient and control the zygoma between the thumb and the intrabuccal index finger of the caudal hand.

The principal technique may be insufficient when there is a post-traumatic impaction. In that situation the practitioner should use the technique described on page 128.

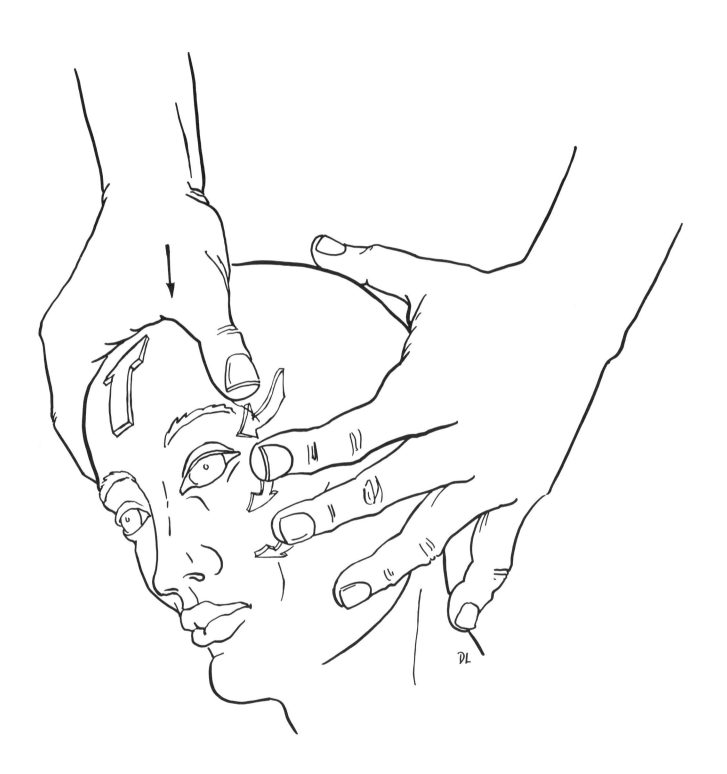

# FRONTOZYGOMATIC DISIMPACTION

**Objective**

To free the articulation between the zygomatic process of the frontal bone and the frontal process of the zygoma from a post-traumatic impaction.

**Position of the patient**

Lying on the side opposite the lesion, comfortable and relaxed. The patient's head is placed on a firm cushion.

**Position of the practitioner**

Standing behind the patient's head, with the treatment table adjusted to a convenient height.

**Points of contact**

The cephalic hand is placed as follows:
—little finger on the greater wing of the sphenoid;
—ring and middle fingers maintain the zygoma in external rotation;
—index finger on the angle of the mandible.
The caudal hand touches the external orbital process of the frontal with its pisiform bone.

**Movement**

While the cephalic hand brings and maintains the zygoma in external rotation, the caudal hand, in accord with all the elements of the so-called "toggle-recoil" technique, performs a thrust. The torque component of this thrust (usually toward the vertex) will be determined by the nature of the impaction.

**Comment**

This technique, which is very effective, is only suitable for practitioners who have attained a high degree of proficiency in the "toggle-recoil" technique.

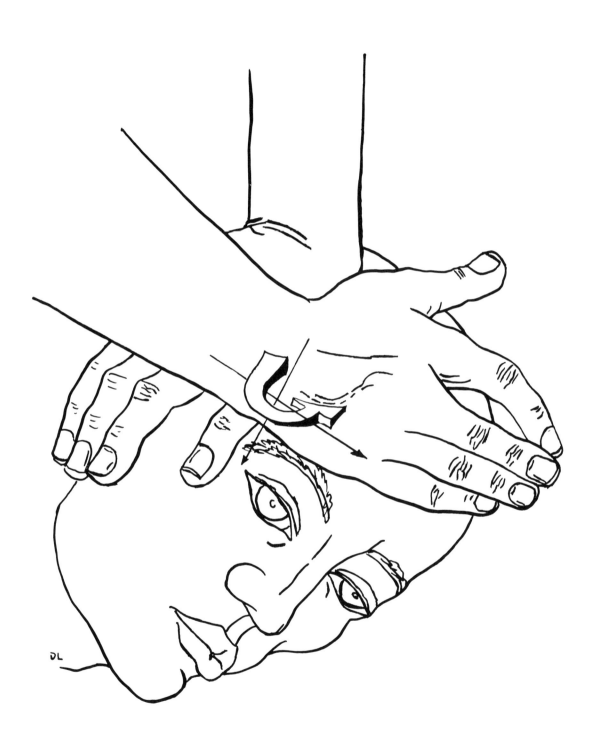

# FRONTOMAXILLARY TECHNIQUE

**Objective**

To free the articulation of the frontal process of the maxilla and the nasal crest of the frontal.

**Position of the patient**

Supine, comfortable and relaxed.

**Position of the practitioner**

Seated at the patient's head, on the side opposite the lesion, with the table adjusted to a convenient height.

**Points of contact**

The cephalic hand controls the frontal bone and the frontal process of the maxilla as follows:
— palm cupping the frontal bone in front of the coronal suture;
— middle finger lodged behind the external orbital process of the frontal bone, on the side of the lesion;
— thumb behind the external orbital process of the frontal bone on the side opposite the lesion;
— pad of the distal phalanx of the index finger touching the superior part of the frontal process of the maxilla.

The index finger of the other hand is intrabuccal and touches the inferior surface of the maxillary apex with its radial edge.

**Movement** (technique applied to the left)

1st phase:  the cephalic hand draws the frontal in flexion during the expansion phase.

2nd phase:  the index finger of the caudal hand, by a lateral rotation around its longitudinal axis, encourages external rotation of the maxilla. The rotation can be increased by slightly lifting the apex of the maxilla with the right index finger, and by disengaging the frontal process caudally in a more coronal plane with the left index finger.

In an acceptable variation, the cephalic hand grasps only the frontal, with the middle finger of the caudal hand intrabuccal and its index finger on the frontal process of the maxilla.

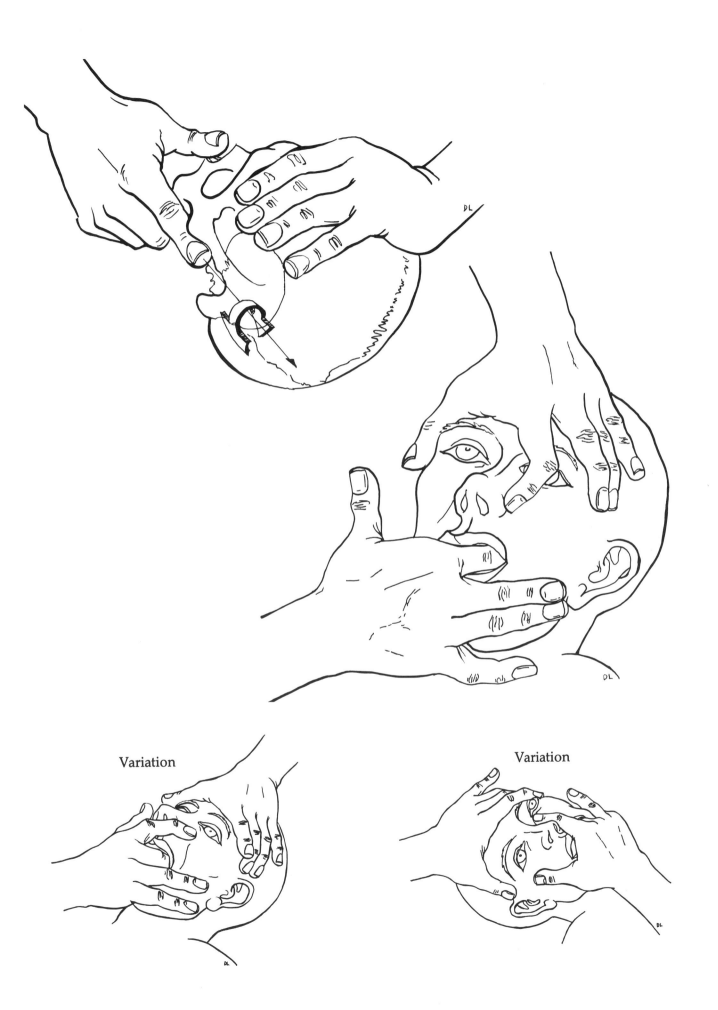

Variation

Variation

# FRONTONASAL TECHNIQUE

**Objective**

To free the articulation of the nasal spine of the frontal and the superior medial border of the nasal bone.

**Position of the patient**

Supine, comfortable and relaxed.

**Position of the practitioner**

Seated either to the right or the left of the patient's head, table adjusted to a convenient height.

**Points of contact**

The cephalic hand controls the frontal bone by cupping the bone in front of the coronal suture in the palm, with the thumb placed on the external orbital process of the practitioner's side, and the index and/or middle fingers positioned behind the other external orbital process.

The index finger and thumb of the other hand touch the nasal bones to the right and left of the nasal crest.

**Movement**

During the expansion phase, the cephalic hand draws the frontal bone in flexion, while the clamp of the thumb and index finger of the caudal hand exerts a medial pressure very close to the internasal suture, which is along the sagittal axis of the body. This facilitates the external displacement of the posterior border.

Always during the same phase of the cranial mechanism, the cephalic hand draws the frontal bone in flexion while the practitioner alternately releases each nasal bone with a lateral pressure accompanied by a slight "comma" motion.

**Comment**

This technique has a number of variations in hand positions that produce identical results.

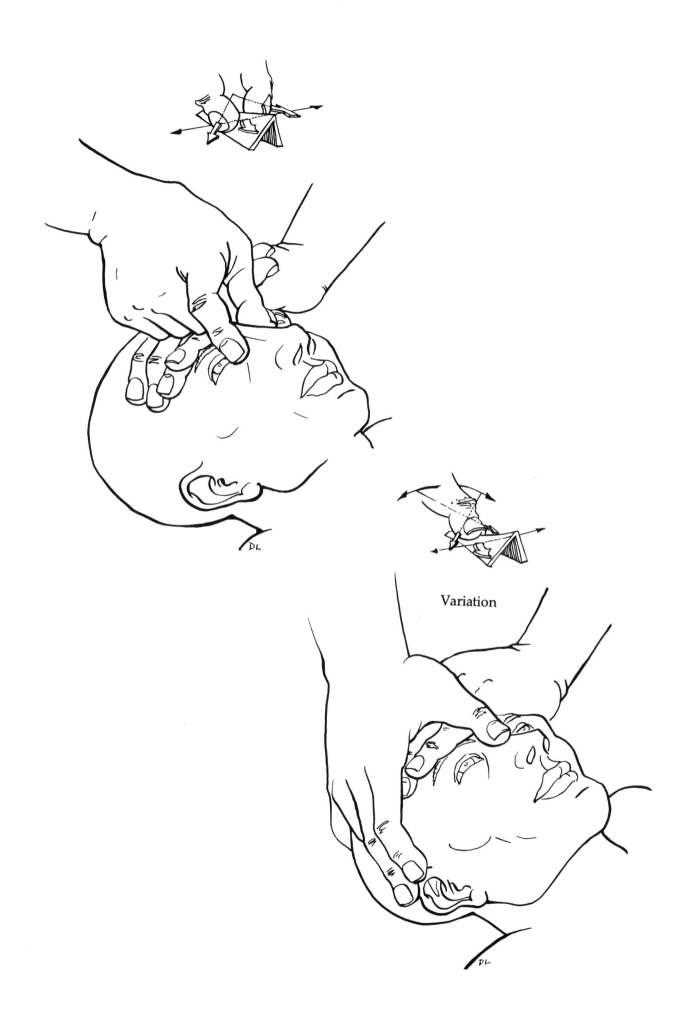

Variation

# FRONTOPARIETAL RELEASE

## Objective

To free the frontoparietal articulation. Near the bregma, the frontal bone is beveled internally, and the parietal externally. Laterally, the bevels are reversed.

## Position of the patient

Supine, comfortable and relaxed.

## Position of the practitioner

Seated at the patient's head on the side opposite the lesion, with the treatment table adjusted to a convenient height.

## Points of contact

The cephalic hand cups the parietal eminence in its palm, and spreads out along the lambda-pterion axis to immobilize the parietal bone on the side of the lesion. The index finger points toward the pterion, the middle finger toward the zygomatic arch of the temporal and the little finger toward the asterion.

The caudal hand, in pronation (with elbow bent), envelops the frontal. The thumb on the practitioner's side, and the little finger on the opposite side, are placed behind the external orbital processes of the frontal.

## Movement

External bevel: during the relaxation phase, the practitioner's caudal hand pulls the lateral aspect of the frontal caudally while simultaneously compressing the external angle of this bone medially so as to increase the release of the parietal.

During the expansion phase, at the same time that the hand on the parietal draws it into external rotation, the practitioner lifts the frontal (in rotation) with the caudal hand.

Internal bevel: during the relaxation phase, the practitioner increases the disengagement of the internal parietal bevel with the cephalic index finger.

As the expansion phase begins, the practitioner draws the parietal in external rotation with the cephalic hand, and lifts the frontal bone in external rotation with the caudal hand.

This cycle is repeated until a release is perceived.

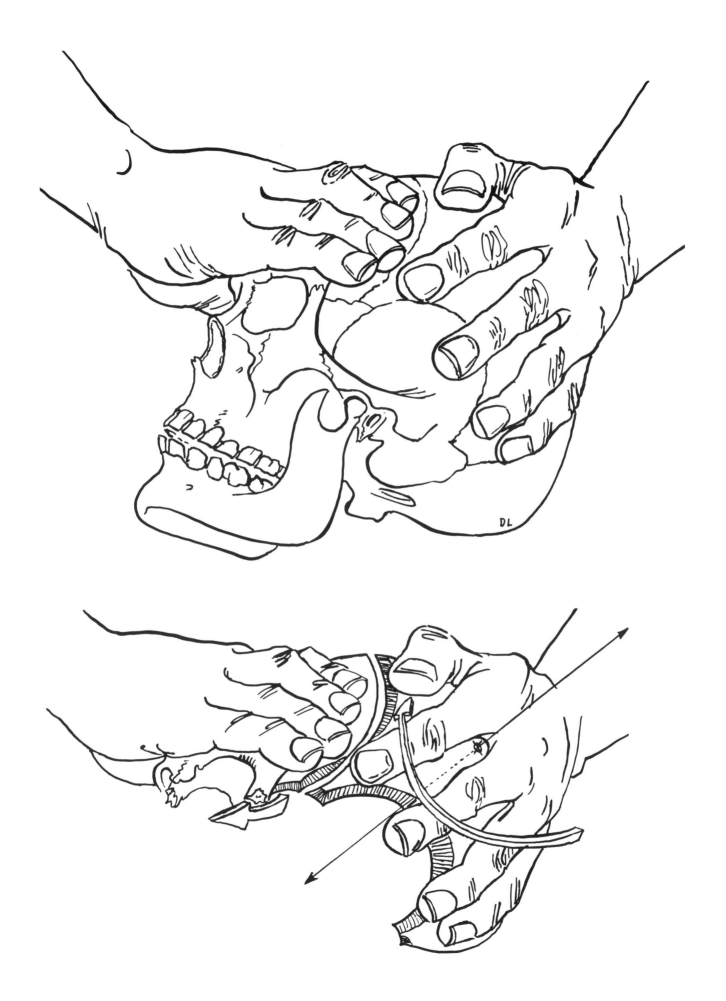

# FRONTOFRONTAL SEPARATION

### Objective

To open a metopic suture which has lost its flexibility either through abnormal development or trauma. This can be done when the frontal bones remain physiologically and functionally apart, or even when the suture has fused. Because the frontal bone always maintains some flexibility along the metopic suture, this technique can be used whenever there is restriction to motion along this suture.

### Position of the patient

Supine, comfortable and relaxed.

### Position of the practitioner

Seated at the patient's head, forearms resting on the treatment table which has been adjusted to a convenient height.

### Points of contact

The thumbs form a "V" pointing caudally, separated by the metopic suture. The other fingers are spread out fan-wise on the frontal bone: index fingers toward the internal orbital process; middle fingers supramedio-orbital; ring fingers placed behind the external orbital process.

Acceptable variations include:

—thumbs interlaced above the metopic suture without touching it;

—index fingers behind the external orbital processes, with other fingers connected.

### Movement

During the expansion phase of the cranial mechanism, while the wrist induces a flexion movement, the fingers draw the frontal bones to let them part at the metopic suture. This is held until a release is perceived.

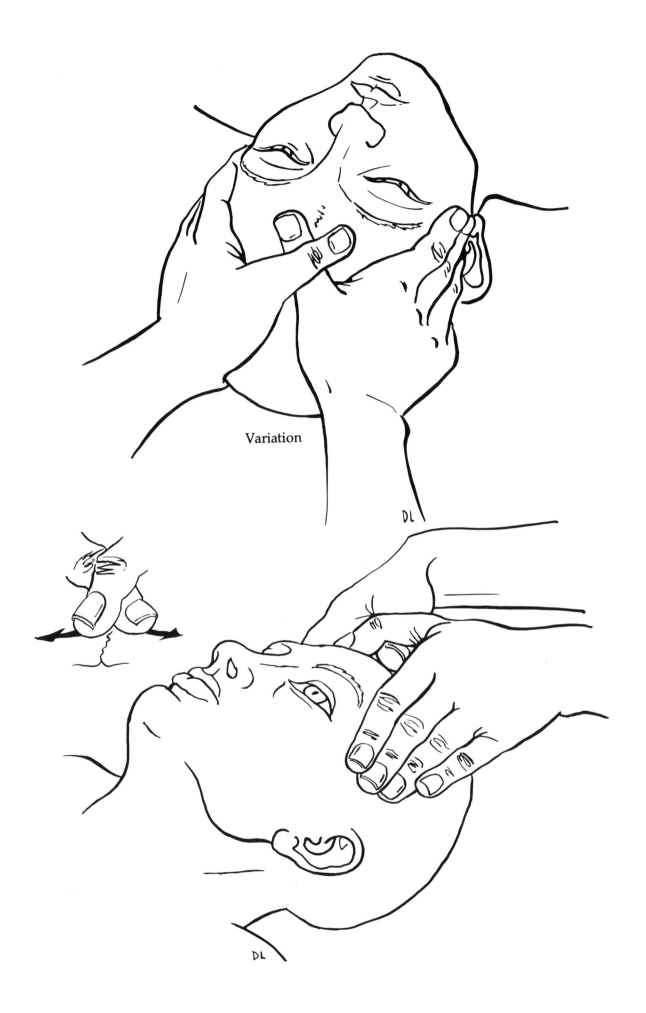

Variation

# V Parietal Techniques

# PARIETAL RELEASE

## Objective

To restore the proper physiological motion to the parietal bones when they are restricted in either internal or external rotation. This technique is normally used as an indirect treatment.

## Position of the patient

Supine, comfortable and relaxed.

## Position of the practitioner

Seated at the patient's head, forearms resting on the treatment table which has been adjusted to a convenient height.

## Points of contact

In a slightly altered vault hold, the practitioner makes the following contacts:
— index fingers on the anteroinferior angles;
— middle fingers immediately above the root of the temporal zygomatic processes;
— ring fingers on the parietomastoid angles;
— thumbs, leaning against each other above the cranium, provide a firm base for the action of the flexor muscles of the fingers.

## Movement

External rotation lesions: the fingers perform a slight disengagement of the external bevels of the parietal by compressing them toward the center of the head during the relaxation phase. The fingers then draw the bone in external rotation during the expansion phase. This is held until a release is perceived.

Internal rotation lesions: after the parietals are disengaged, they are drawn into internal rotation, still during the relaxation phase.

## Comment

These manipulations are performed bilaterally. If the lesion is unilateral, the practitioner's action will be intensified on the side of the lesion. But the integration of the movement of both parietal bones in the movement as a whole is essential. If a serious impaction exists, it is preferable that the therapist choose one of the more powerful manipulative techniques described later in this chapter.

140

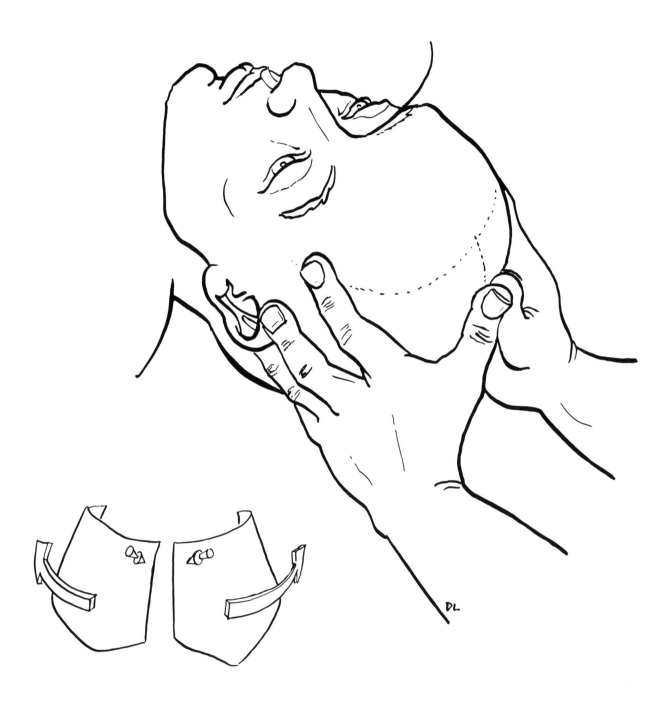

# PARIETAL LIFT

## Objective

To lift the parietal and free it from neighboring bones. This technique is intended to affect circulation.

## Position of the patient

Supine, comfortable and relaxed.

## Position of the practitioner

Seated at the patient's head, forearms resting on the treatment table which has been adjusted to a convenient height. The practitioner holds the patient's head in his or her hands.

## Points of contact

In a slightly altered vault hold, the practitioner makes the following contacts:
— index fingers on the anteroinferior angles;
— middle fingers immediately above the base of the temporal zygomatic processes;
— ring fingers on the parietomastoid angles;
— thumbs, crossed above the sagittal suture, each touching the opposite parietal.

## Movement

1st phase: (Disengagement.) During the relaxation phase, the practitioner's fingers, at the external bevels, press medially to part the parietal from the greater wing of the sphenoid and from the temporal squama by exaggerating the internal rotation of the bone.

2nd phase: (External rotation.) During the expansion phase of the cranial mechanism, the practitioner lifts the parietals in external rotation.

3rd phase: (Lifting.) While continuing the 2nd phase, the parietals are lifted toward the practitioner. This position is held until a release is perceived.

Multiple digital contacts allow for selective release of the lesioned area. Fingers may be placed as follows: index finger on the greater wing and parietal; middle finger on the squamous suture; and ring fingers on the parietomastoid angles.

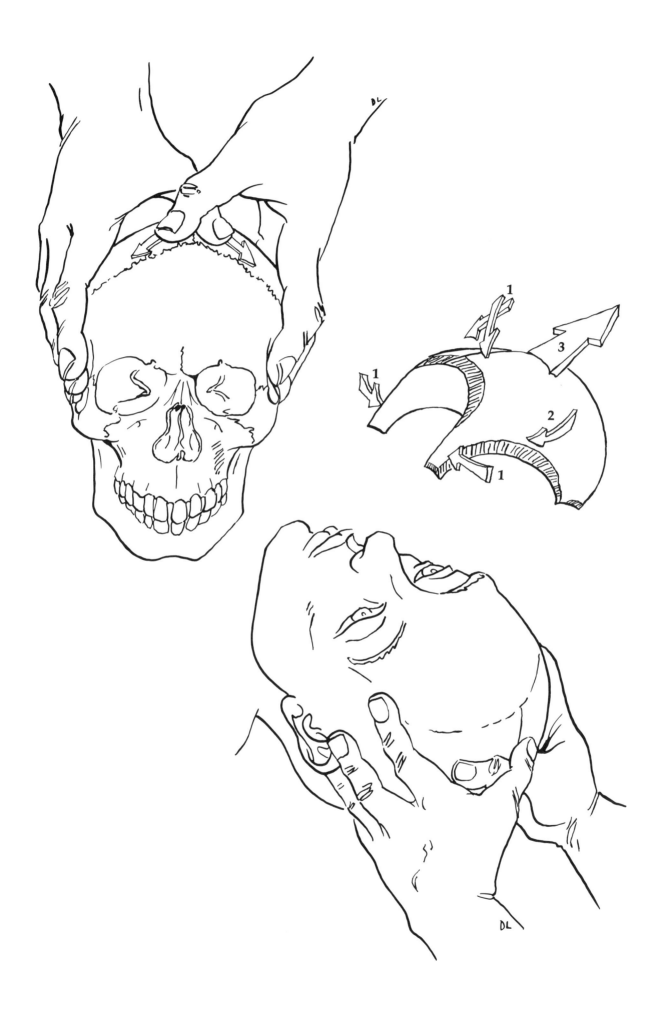

# EXPANSION OF THE PARIETAL

## Objective

To regularize the circulation in the longitudinal sinuses, and to harmonize the relationship between the tentorium and the falx.

## Position of the patient

Supine, comfortable and relaxed.

## Position of the practitioner

Seated at the patient's head, forearms resting on the treatment table which has been adjusted to a convenient height. The practitioner holds the patient's head in his or her hands.

## Points of contact

In a slightly altered vault hold, the practitioner makes the following contacts:
— index fingers on the squamous borders of the parietals;
— ring fingers on the mastoid processes;
— thumbs, crossed above the sagittal suture, in the posteroinferior angles of the parietals, as close as possible to the lambda.

## Movement

Only the thumbs are active; the other fingers simply hold the patient's head steady.

During the expansion phase, the practitioner exerts pressure with the thumbs toward the vertex and anteriorly to part the parietals from the occipital, and also laterally, drawing the thumbs away from each other. The pressure is released at the beginning of the relaxation phase. This process is repeated until a release is perceived.

## Comment

When there is an impaction this technique is often insufficient; the technique for disimpaction of the lambda must be used instead (page 146).

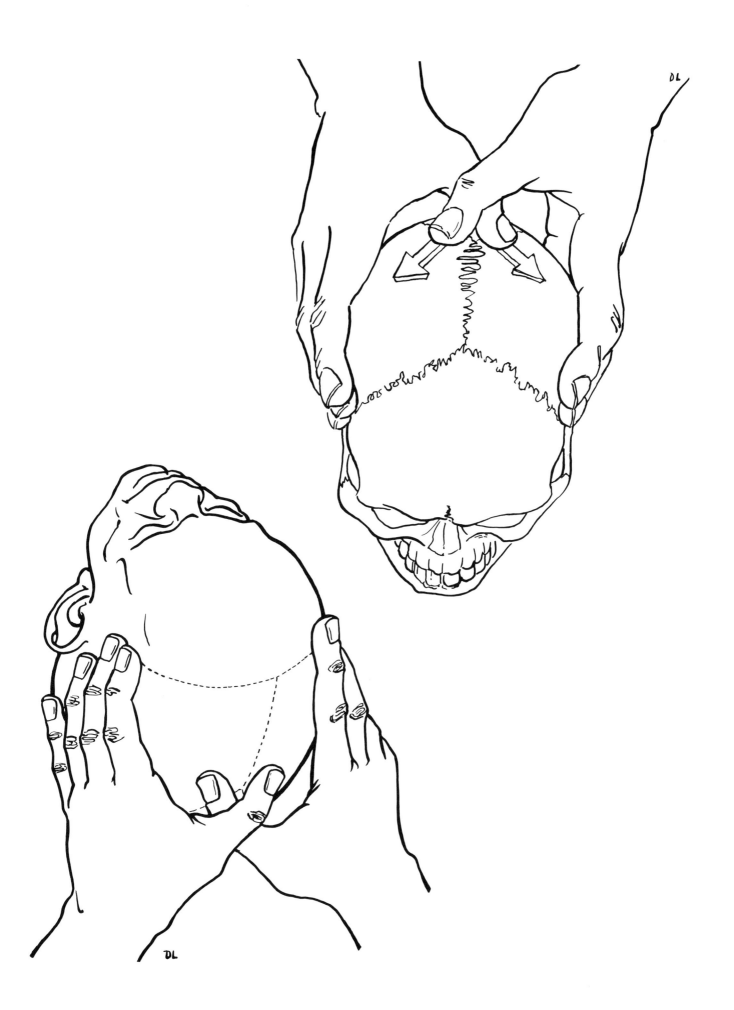

# DISIMPACTION OF THE LAMBDA

### Objective

To restore normal functional freedom to the lambda, the meeting place of the sagittal and lambdoid sutures.

### Position of the patient

Supine, comfortable and relaxed.

### Position of the practitioner

Seated at the patient's head, forearms resting on the treatment table which has been adjusted to a convenient height.

### Points of contact

In a slightly altered vault hold, the practitioner makes the following digital contacts:
— little fingers (forming a "V" and making contact with the tips of their distal phalanges) on the superior portion of the occipital squama, close to the lambda;
— ring fingers just lateral to the sagittal suture;
— middle fingers immediately above the zygomatic process;
— index fingers on the anteroinferior angle of the parietals.

The crossed thumbs are situated as close as possible to the lambda, each one on the posterosuperior angle of the opposite parietal.

### Movement

During the relaxation phase, the thumbs disengage the parietal angles by pressing them toward the center of the head.

When the expansion phase begins, the little fingers accentuate the flexion of the occiput. At the same time, the thumbs draw the posteroinferior angles of the parietals toward the vertex while trying to part them from each other. The other fingers lead the parietals into external rotation.

### Comment

This technique can be performed with the patient seated and the practitioner standing behind.

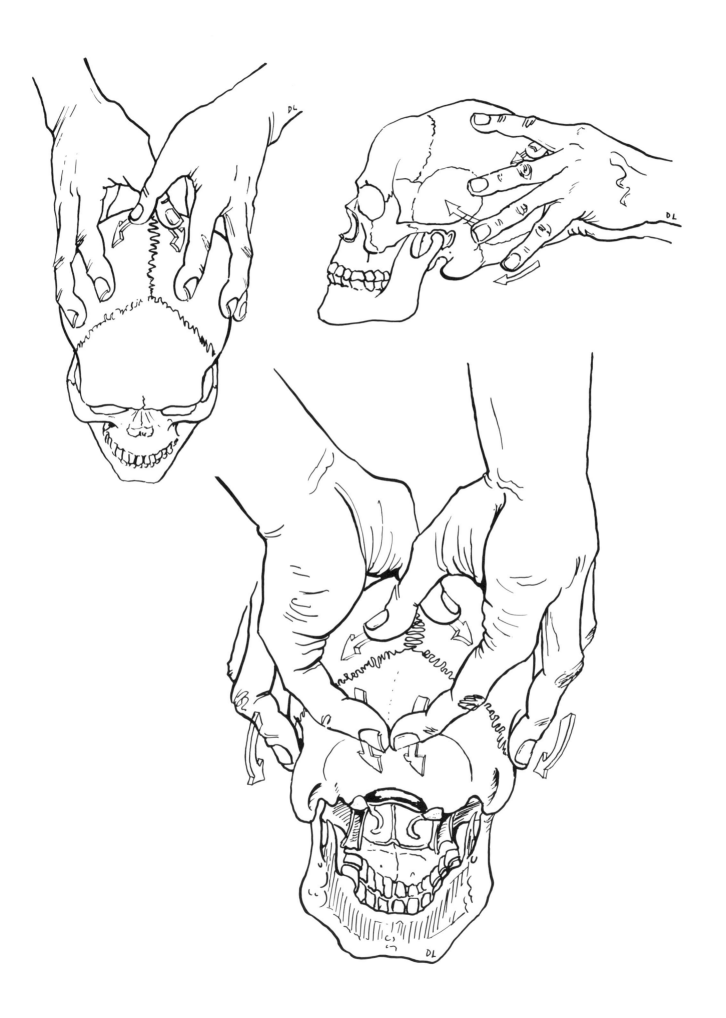

# POSTERIOR INTERPARIETAL SUTURAL OPENING

**Objective**

To open the posterior portion of the sagittal suture.

**Position of the patient**

Supine, comfortable and relaxed.

**Position of the practitioner**

Seated at the patient's head, forearms resting on the treatment table which has been adjusted to a convenient height. The practitioner holds the patient's head in his or her hands.

**Points of contact**

In this vault hold, the index fingers are placed on the anteroinferior angles of the parietals, with the middle fingers immediately above the root of the zygomatic process of the temporal. The ring fingers are on the parietomastoid angles. The thumbs are crossed above the sagittal suture; each one touches the opposite parietal along its lambdoid border, as close as possible to the lambda.

**Movement**

This technique is performed in three smoothly-linked phases: the first during the relaxation phase, and the other two during the expansion phase.

1st phase:   (Release.) The practitioner presses on the parietals in order to free them from the occiput.

2nd phase:   (Opening.) The practitioner opens the posterior part of the interparietal sagittal suture by drawing the thumbs apart from each other.

3rd phase:   (External rotation.) The other fingers, spread out on the cranium, encourage external rotation of the parietals.

**Comment**

In order to disengage the overlapping surfaces the practitioner may, during the 2nd phase, draw the thumbs apart while scrupulously respecting the palpable direction of the sutural force lines.

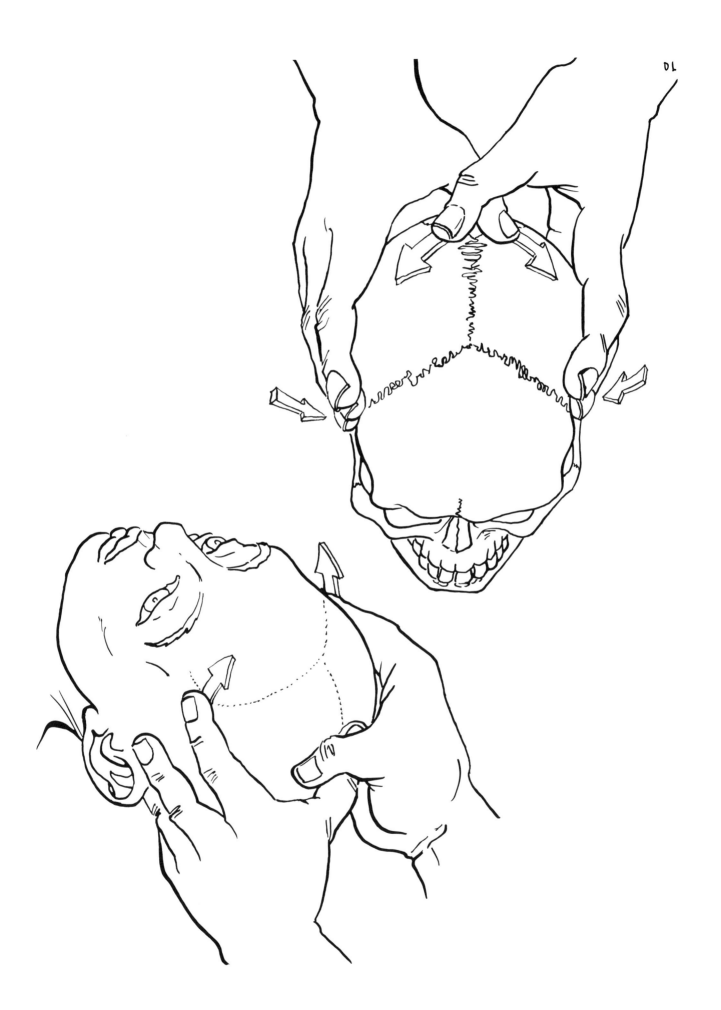

# INTERPARIETAL SUTURAL OPENING

## Objective

To restore functional freedom at the indentations of the sagittal suture.

## Position of the patient

Supine, comfortable and relaxed.

## Position of the practitioner

Seated at the patient's head, forearms resting on the treatment table which has been adjusted to a convenient height. The practitioner holds the patient's head in his or her hands.

## Points of contact

The thumbs are placed parallel to each side of the sagittal suture from the bregma. The other fingers are spread out on the squama of the parietals.

## Movement

During the expansion phase, the thumbs draw apart slightly from each other while the other fingers accentuate the external rotation movement of the parietals.

The practitioner should be especially forceful where he or she has felt restriction of mobility during the examination.

In order to have a definite effect, it is important to pay close attention to the subtleties of the direction of release of the sutural indentations.

## Comment

This technique can be performed with the patient seated on the edge of the treatment table, and the practitioner standing behind.

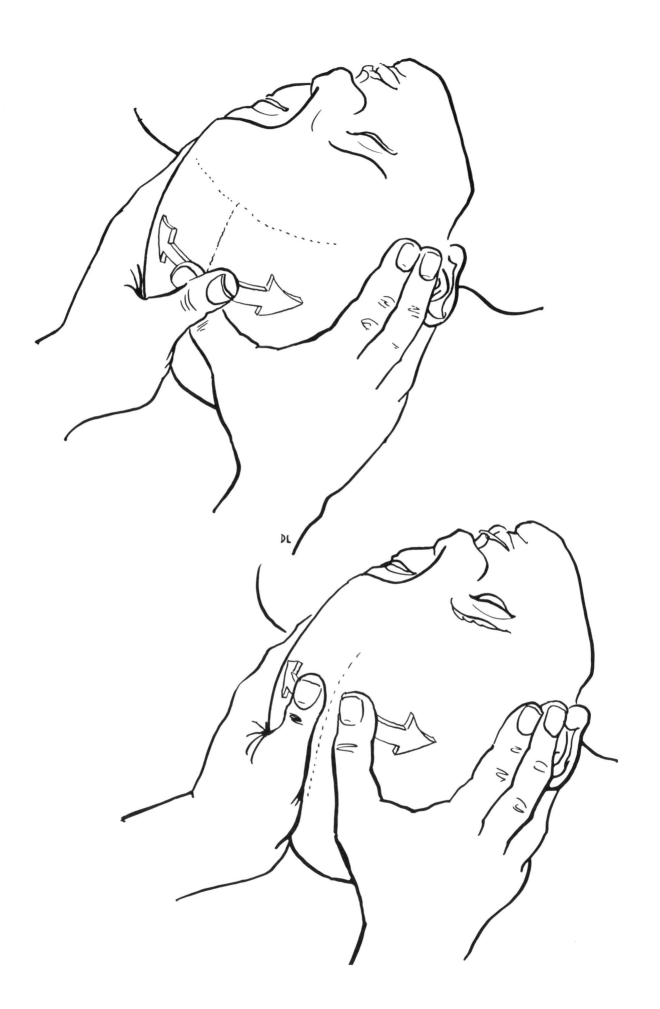

# PARIETOFRONTAL DISENGAGEMENT

## LATERAL ASPECT

### Objective

To restore articular functional freedom, when trauma has resulted in a compression of the frontal bone between the parietals.

### Position of the patient

Sitting on the edge of the treatment table, which has been adjusted to a rather low height.

### Position of the practitioner

Standing and facing the patient, elbows bent, with the interlaced fingers of both hands covering the patient's cranium.

### Points of contact

The thenar eminences are placed on the lateral aspect of the parietals, close to the pterions. The hypothenar eminences are positioned on the squama. The other fingers are interlaced above the sagittal suture.

### Movement

During the relaxation phase of cranial motion, using the flexor muscles of the fingers, the practitioner compresses both parietals medially, disengaging them from the frontal.

During the expansion phase, the practitioner lifts the parietals toward the vertex while maintaining all digital contacts.

### Comment

The description above is of the technique for the lateral aspect of the parietofrontal suture only. For medial lesions close to the bregma, the practitioner should apply the technique described on page 154.

If there is a unilateral lesion, the frontoparietal technique on page 134 should be employed.

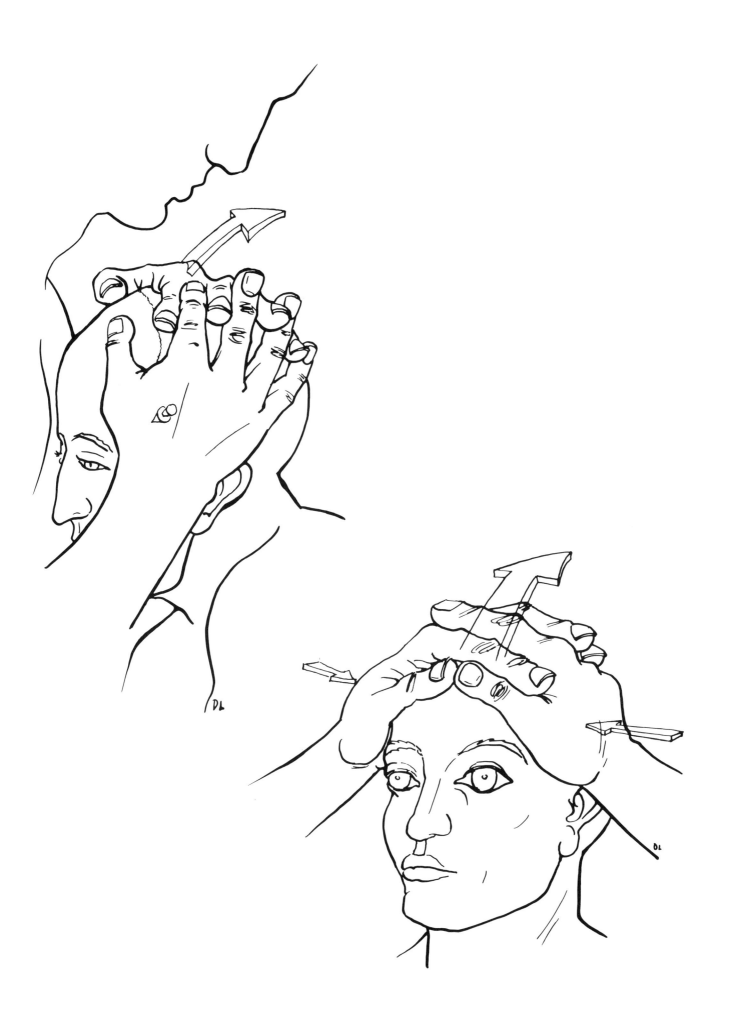

# DISIMPACTION OF THE BREGMA

### Objective

To restore physiological functional freedom to the bregma, the meeting place of the sagittal and coronal sutures.

### Position of the patient

Supine, comfortable and relaxed.

### Position of the practitioner

Seated at the patient's head, forearms resting on the treatment table which has been adjusted to a convenient height.

### Points of contact

In a slightly altered vault hold, the practitioner makes the following digital contacts:
— index fingers placed behind the external orbital processes of the frontal;
— thumbs, crossed above the anterior sagittal suture, placed on the anterosuperior angle of the opposite parietal;
— ring fingers on the mastoid angles of the parietals.

### Movement

The disengagement is achieved during the relaxation phase by pressure of the thumbs on the parietals.

During the expansion phase, the index fingers accompany the flexion of the frontal and draw it in a slightly anterior direction. The thumbs, while moving apart, push the anterosuperior angles of the parietals in a posterior direction, while the ring fingers accentuate the external rotation of those bones. This is held until a release is perceived.

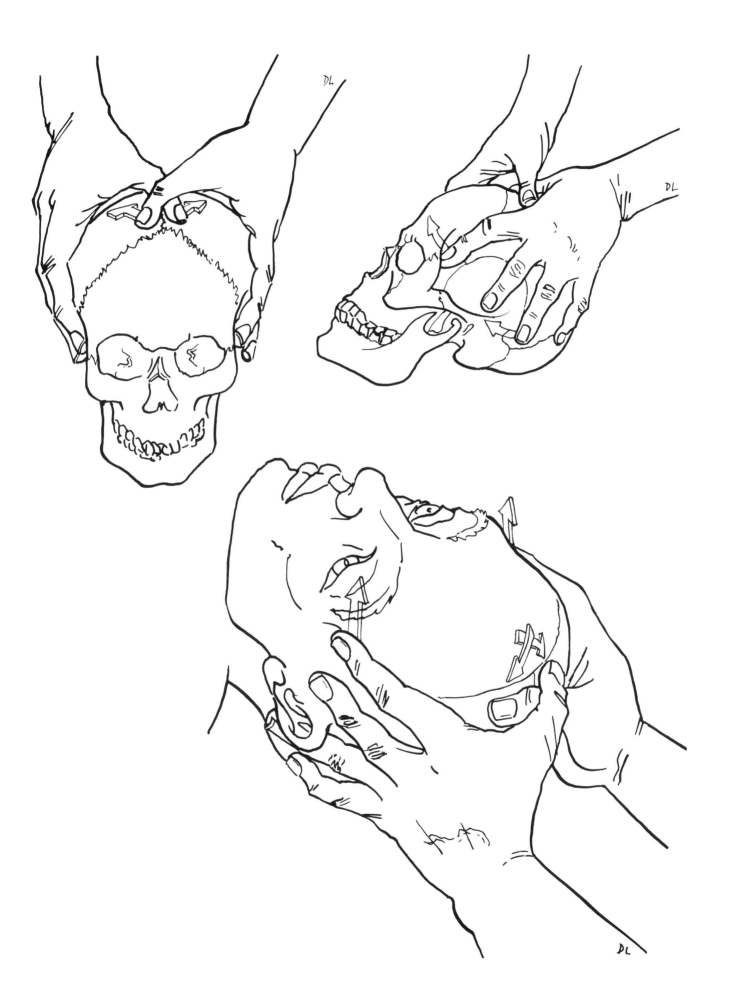

# SPHENOPARIETAL DISENGAGEMENT

## BILATERAL

### Objective

To restore functional freedom to the sphenoparietal articulation, particularly when it has been affected by trauma in the anterosuperior parts of the parietals.

### Position of the patient

Sitting on the edge of the treatment table, which has been adjusted to a rather low height.

### Position of the practitioner

Standing and facing the patient, elbows bent, the fingers of both hands interlaced and covering the patient's cranium.

### Points of contact

The thenar eminences are placed on the sphenoidal angles of the parietals. The hypothenar eminences are placed further along, on the squama of the parietals. The other fingers are interlaced and positioned above the sagittal suture.

### Movement

During the relaxation phase of cranial motion, the flexor muscles of the practitioner's fingers compress the sphenoidal angles of the parietals medially.

During the expansion phase, the practitioner lifts the parietals toward the vertex while maintaining all digital contacts. The position of balanced tension is held until a release is perceived.

### Comment

This is a variation of the technique described on page 152.

Although it is possible to perform this technique unilaterally, working on one side only and simply maintaining the other side, this often proves to be ineffective. It is preferable to utilize the technique described on page 158 when there is a unilateral lesion.

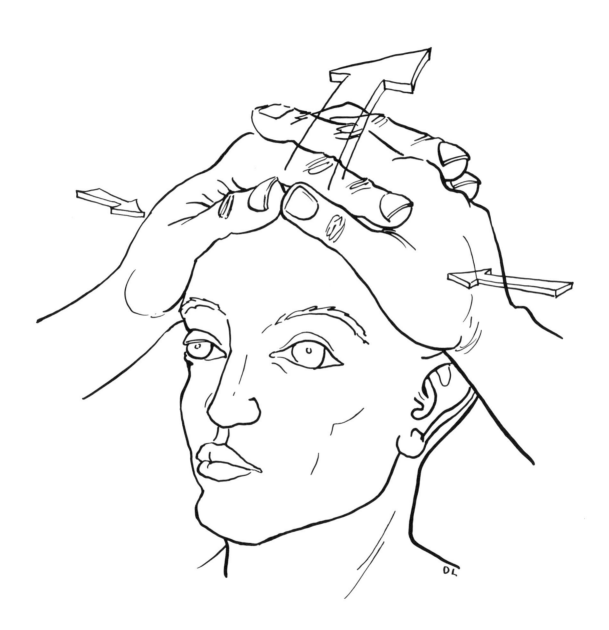

# SPHENOPARIETAL DISENGAGEMENT

## UNILATERAL

### Objective

To restore functional freedom to the sphenoparietal articulation when it has been unilaterally altered as a consequence of trauma on the anterior part of the parietal bone.

### Position of the patient

Supine, comfortable and relaxed.

### Position of the practitioner

Seated at the patient's head on the side opposite the lesion, the table adjusted to a convenient height.

### Points of contact

The caudal hand controls the sphenoid as follows:
— clamp of the thumb and index finger enveloping the frontal bone and ending on the greater wings;
— little finger, intrabuccal, placed on the external surface of the pterygoid process.

The cephalic hand makes the following parietal contacts:
— thumb placed along the coronal suture;
— index finger at the sphenoid angle;
— other fingers spread out on the squama.

### Movement

During the relaxation phase of cranial motion, the index finger of the cephalic hand compresses the sphenoid angle of the parietal medially to disengage it.

During the expansion phase, each hand follows the external rotation of the bone it controls to its respective limit while drawing apart from the other hand. This maneuver is continued until a release is perceived.

### Comment

To be effective, the execution of this rather energetic technique must scrupulously respect the progressive relaxation of the periarticular tissues.

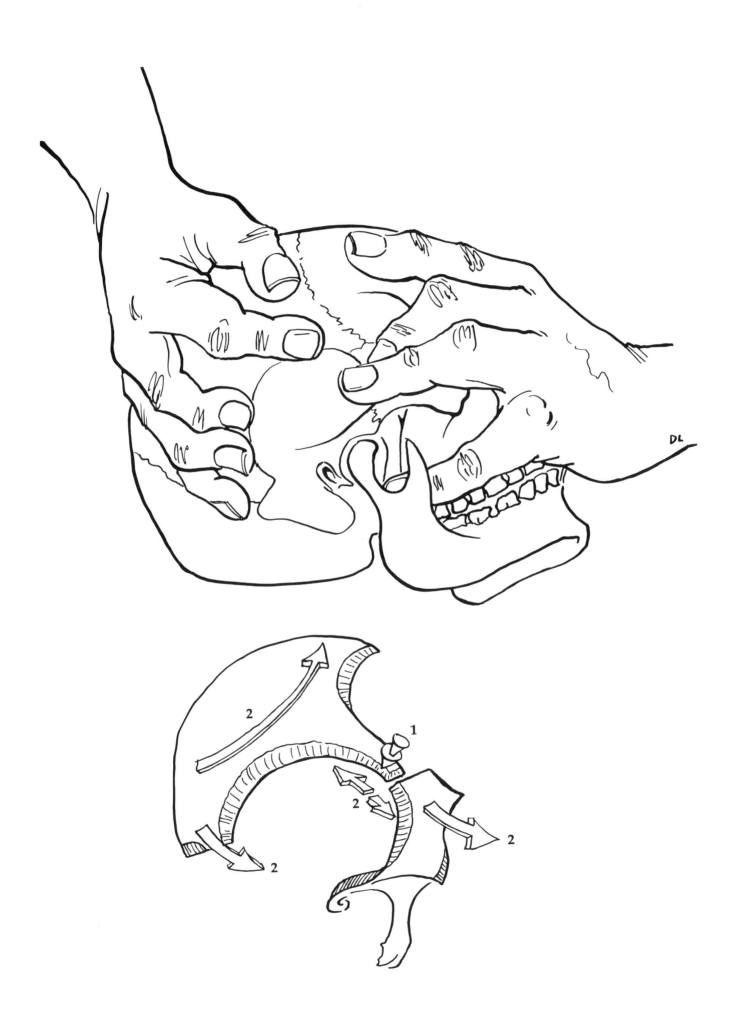

# PARIETO-OCCIPITAL DISENGAGEMENT

### Objective

To restore functional freedom of the parieto-occipital articulation, the bones of which have been forced into each other after a caudal shift of the posteroinferior angles of the parietals as a result of trauma in the lambdoid area.

### Position of the patient

Sitting on the edge of the treatment table, which has been adjusted to a rather low height.

### Position of the practitioner

Standing behind the patient, elbows bent, the fingers of both hands interlaced and crowning the posterior portions of the patient's cranium.

### Points of contact

The practitioner positions the thenar eminences on the posteroinferior angles of the parietals. The fingers are interlaced above the sagittal suture, with the index fingers as close to the lambdoid suture as possible.

### Movement

During the relaxation phase of the cranial mechanism, the practitioner compresses the posteroinferior angles of the parietals medially, while disengaging the occiput.

During the expansion phase, the practitioner lifts the parietals slightly toward the vertex, while simultaneously pronating the forearms to accentuate the external rotation of the bones. This is continued until a release is perceived.

### Comment

The description above is for a bilateral lesion. When there is a unilateral lesion, only one angle is actually compressed; the other is simply held in position.

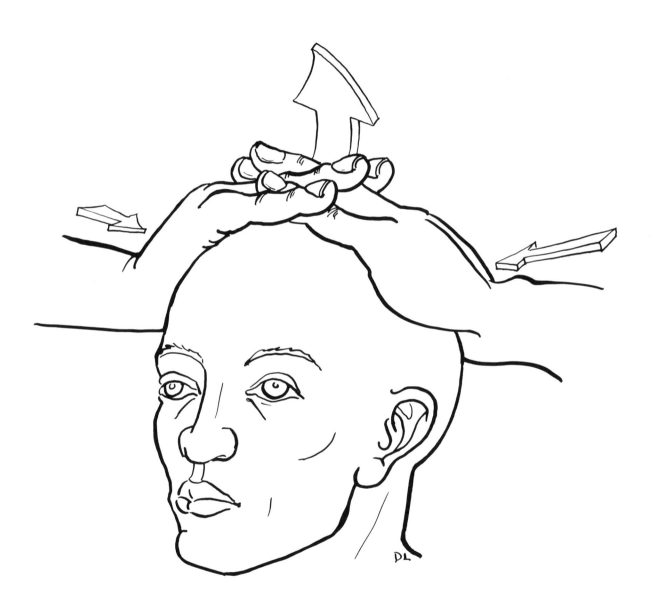

# TEMPOROPARIETAL DISENGAGEMENT

### Objective

To restore functional freedom to the temporoparietal suture.

### Position of the patient

Supine, comfortable and relaxed.

### Position of the practitioner

Seated at the patient's head, forearms resting on the treatment table which has been adjusted to a convenient height. The practitioner holds the patient's head in his or her hands.

### Points of contact

The practitioner's hands, in a modified vault hold, make the following symmetrical contacts on each side of the patient's cranium:

— heads of the metacarpals on the parietal portion of the squamous suture;

— index fingers on the zygomatic processes of the temporals;

— little fingers on the anterior part of the mastoid processes.

### Movement

During the relaxation phase of cranial motion, the heads of the metacarpals compress the parietal part of the squamous suture medially.

During the expansion phase, the index and ring fingers exaggerate the external rotation of the temporals. At the same time, both hands of the practitioner, with a continuous action of the heads of the metacarpals, lift the parietals in the direction of the vertex, disengaging the squamous suture.

### Comment

In the case of a unilateral lesion, only one hand is active; the other simply maintains its position.

The functional freedom of the temporomandibular joint must be ensured, since any traumatic impaction here tends to produce a secondary lesion of the temporoparietal suture.

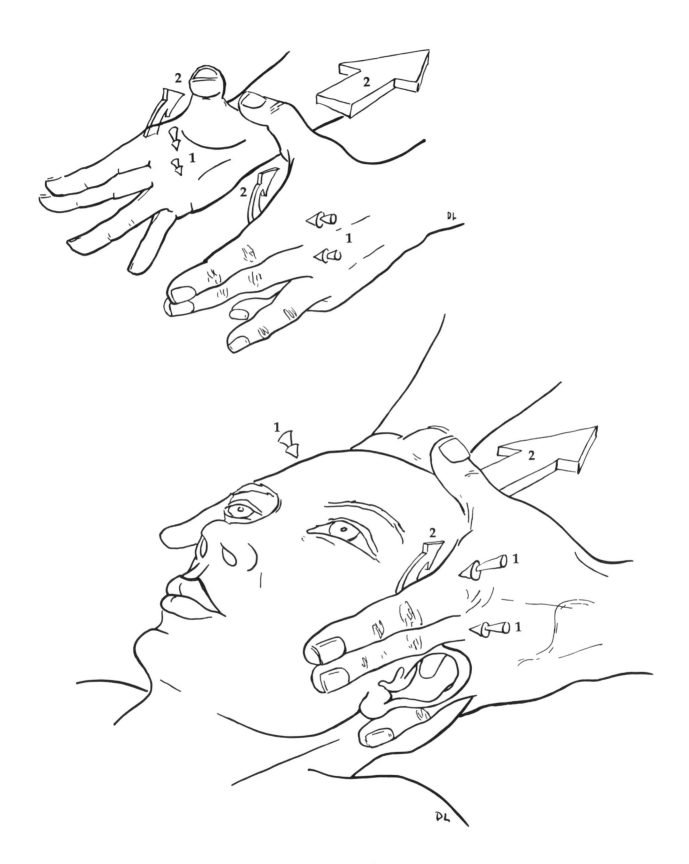

# UNILATERAL DISENGAGEMENT
# OF THE DEEP POSTEROINFERIOR ANGLE

**Objective**

To unilaterally disengage the posteroinferior angle (parietomastoid suture).

**Position of the patient**

Supine, comfortable and relaxed.

**Position of the practitioner**

Seated at the patient's head, forearms resting on the treatment table which has been adjusted to a convenient height.

**Points of contact**

The interlaced fingers of the practitioner's supine hands hold the posterior part of the cranium. On the side of the lesion, the thenar eminence is placed on the posteroinferior angle of the parietal. On the other side, it touches the lateral angle of the occipital squama. The thumbs are spread out along the corresponding mastoid processes.

**Movement**

During the relaxation phase of cranial motion, both thenar eminences exert a gentle and constant pressure toward the center of the cranium.

During the expansion phase, both thumbs draw the tip of the mastoid processes in a posterior and medial direction (external rotation). At the same time, the thenar eminence moves the posteroinferior angle of the corresponding parietal in an anterior and cephalad direction.

This technique is repeated until the practitioner perceives a release by way of relaxation of the tissues. The relaxation accompanies a permanent disengagement of this angle.

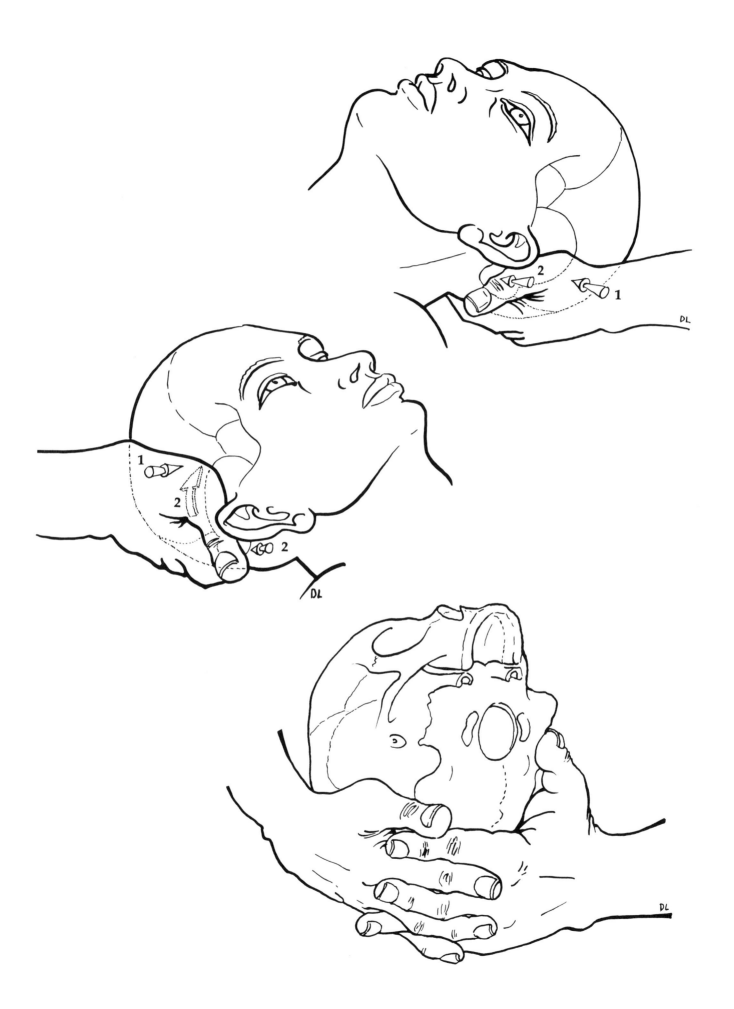

# VI  Sphenoidal Techniques

The manipulative techniques for the bones of the base and the vault have been described. Those involving the sphenobasilar joint have been dealt with, for the most part, in the introductory section of general techniques that have a direct influence upon the cranial mechanism as a whole. Here, we will describe two particularly effective techniques for the sphenoid.

# REPOSITIONING OF THE SPHENOID

**Objective**

To restore functional freedom between the sphenoid and the occiput.

**Position of the patient**

Supine, comfortable and relaxed.

**Position of the practitioner**

Seated beside the treatment table, facing the patient's head. The treatment table has been adjusted to a rather low height, so that the patient's head is level with the practitioner's hands.

**Points of contact**

The cephalic hand cradles the occiput from the lambda to the inion along the longitudinal axis of the hand.

The caudal hand controls the sphenoid as follows:
— the clamp of the thumb and index finger facing the frontal without making contact;
— terminal phalanges of the thumb and index finger on the greater wings;
— intrabuccal little finger on the pterygoid process.

**Movement**

During the expansion phase of cranial motion, the cephalic hand draws the occiput in flexion. As this occurs, the caudal hand positions the sphenoid on its three axes (anteroposterior, transverse and vertical) in order to reach the point of balance which permits the physiological movement of the synchondrosis. The point of balanced tension is maintained until a release is perceived.

**Comment**

This technique is particularly effective because it utilizes excellent control of the sphenoid. Its one drawback is that it demands a high level of precision in the movements of the cephalic hand.

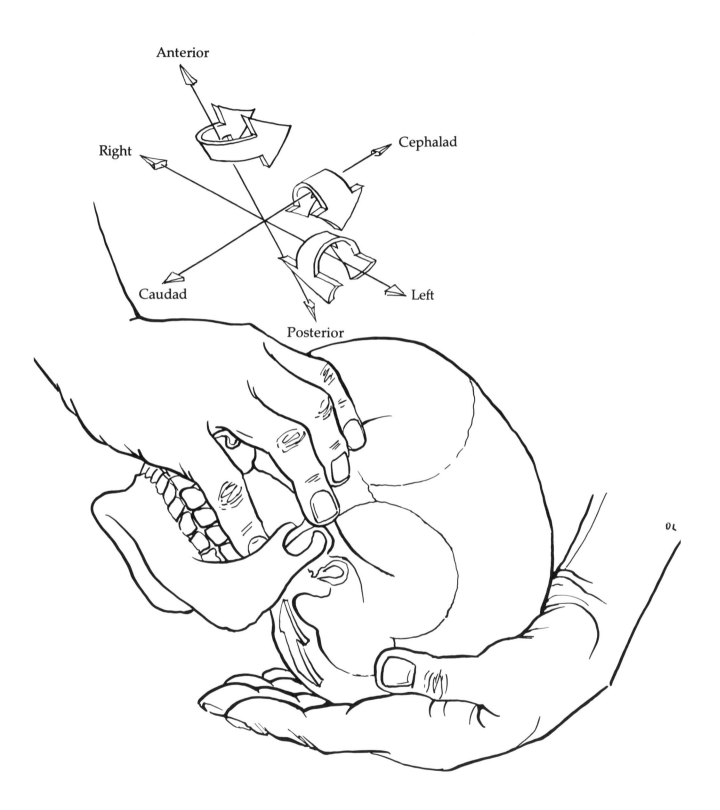

# DRAINAGE OF THE SPHENOIDAL SINUS

**Objective**

To cause the drainage of purulent secretions that have been abnormally retained in the sphenoidal sinus.

**Position of the patient**

Supine, comfortable and relaxed.

**Position of the practitioner**

Seated beside the treatment table, facing the patient's head. The table has been adjusted to a convenient height.

**Points of contact**

The cephalic hand controls the sphenoid as follows:
—the clamp of thumb and index finger span the frontal bone without making contact;
—the terminal phalanges of thumb and index finger placed on the greater wings.

The index finger of the caudal hand is placed on the palate beneath the cruciate suture, establishing a firm base for manipulation.

**Movement**

The practitioner's hands perform an oppositional movement.

During the expansion phase of cranial motion, the cephalic hand draws the sphenoid in flexion, while the intraoral index finger opposes the thrust of the vomer (at the cruciate suture) with a pressure toward the body of the sphenoid.

During the relaxation phase, there is a return to the neutral position; the practitioner's hands are passive. This cycle is continued until a release is perceived.

**Comment**

It is still necessary to treat the primary or causal lesions in these cases.

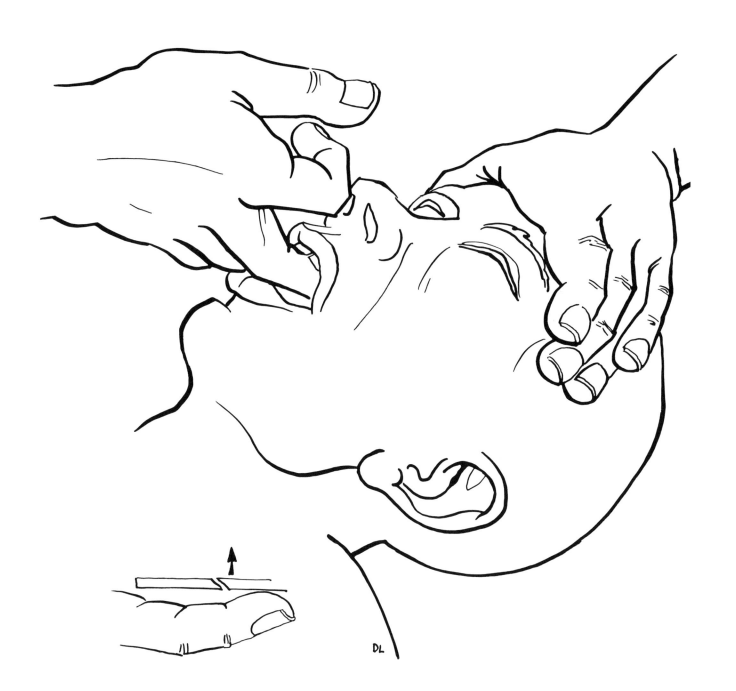

# VII    Facial Bones

# GENERAL FACIAL RELEASE

## FIRST TECHNIQUE

### Objective

To harmonize the functional relationship of all the bones of the face during the motions of external and internal rotation.

### Position of the patient

Supine, comfortable and relaxed.

### Position of the practitioner

Seated at the patient's head, forearms resting on the treatment table which has been adjusted to a convenient height. The practitioner holds the patient's head in his or her hands.

### Points of contact

The palms of the hands lie on the frontal surface so that both thumbs, forming a "V", join on the metopic suture near the glabella.

The index and middle fingers are spread out on the patient's cheeks and frame the external surface of the maxillae.

### Movement

During the expansion phase of cranial motion, the palms of the hands and the thumbs initiate an external rotation of the frontal bone, while the middle and index fingers carry along the maxillae. The resultant point of balanced tension is maintained until a release is perceived.

This technique can also be performed during internal rotation.

### Comment

This technique must be applied very gently and should be repeated several times in a row so that the motion of each facial bone is completely integrated into the general motion of the cranium. This will require multiple releases.

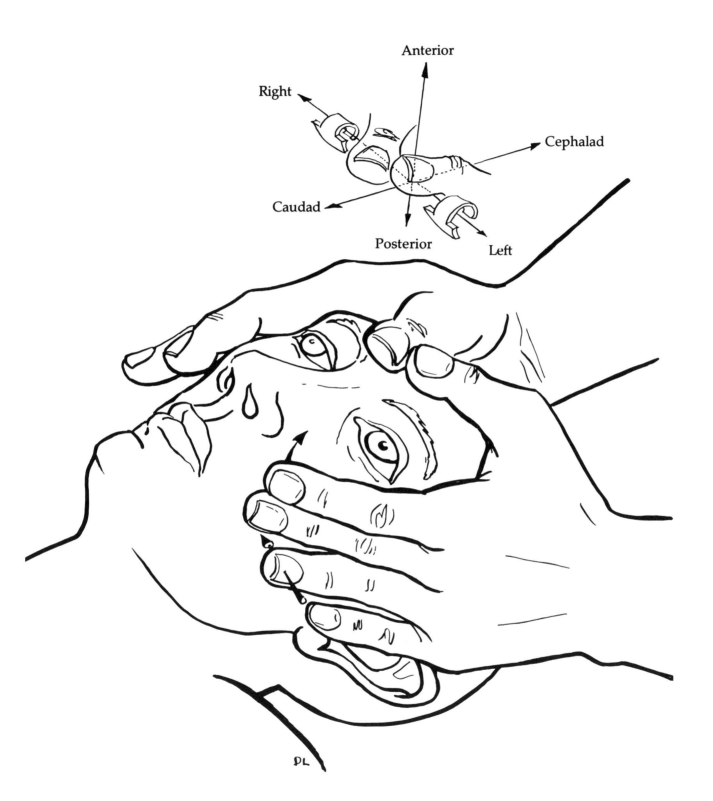

# GENERAL FACIAL RELEASE

## SECOND TECHNIQUE

### Objective

To harmonize the functional relationship of all the facial bones during the motions of external and internal rotation.

### Position of the patient

Supine, comfortable and relaxed.

### Position of the practitioner

Seated at the patient's head, on the side opposite the lesion, the table adjusted to a convenient height.

### Points of contact

The cephalic hand is positioned over the frontal bone, with the thumb and the index or middle finger on the greater wings of the sphenoid.

On the caudal hand, the intraoral index finger touches the palate at the cruciate suture.

### Movement

During the expansion phase of cranial motion, the cephalic hand draws the greater wings of the sphenoid in a caudal and anterior direction. Simultaneously, the palm, by a slight supination, initiates the flexion of the frontal. The index finger of the other hand accentuates this movement by exerting a gentle and constant pressure toward the base of the nose.

During the relaxation phase, the frontal hand, while bringing this bone in internal rotation, draws the greater wings cephalad and posteriorly. At the same time, the intraoral index finger pushes the cruciate suture cephalad, toward the body of the sphenoid.

This sequence is repeated until a release is perceived.

### Comment

This technique must be applied very gently and should be repeated several times so that the motion of each facial bone is completely integrated into the general motion of the cranium. This will require multiple releases.

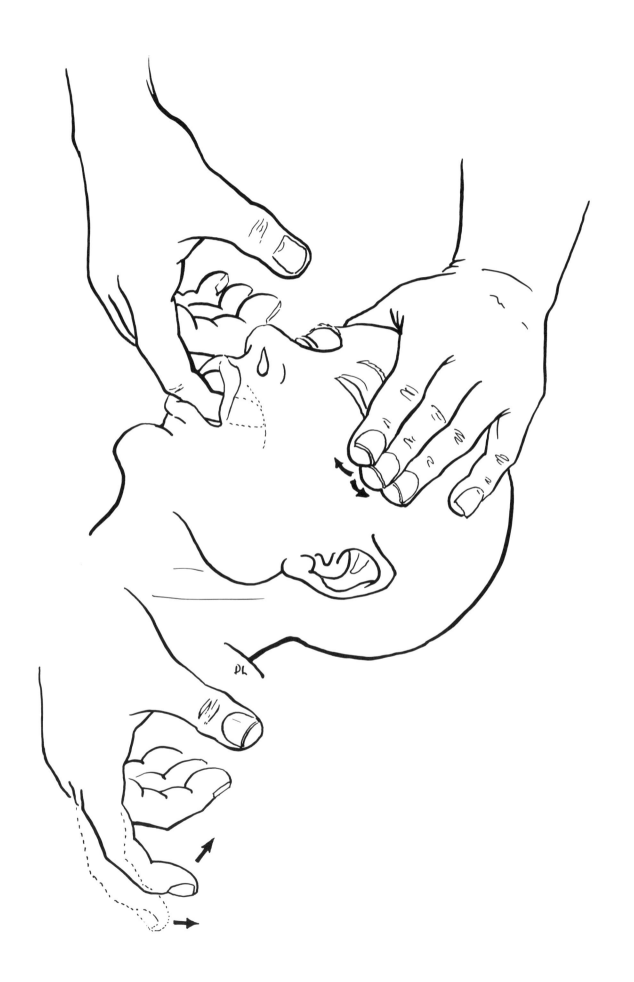

# BALANCING OF THE MAXILLA WITH THE ZYGOMA

## Objective

To reestablish the physiological mobility of the maxilla in the general motion of the cranium.

## Position of the patient

Supine, comfortable and relaxed.

## Position of the practitioner

Seated at the patient's head, forearms resting on the treatment table which has been adjusted to a convenient height. The practitioner holds the patient's head in his or her hands.

## Points of contact

The practitioner's thumbs touch the zygomae, while the index and middle fingers are hooked beneath the horizontal ridges of the maxillae.

## Movement

During the expansion phase of cranial motion, the thumbs induce external rotation of the zygomae laterally and caudally. Simultaneously, the fingers move the maxillae into a more coronal plane, shifting the horizontal ridges externally with the mid-incisor line moving back slightly. This is external rotation of the maxillae.

During the relaxation phase, the practitioner's hands are passive. This cycle is repeated until a release is perceived.

In an acceptable variation, the fingers hooked under the maxillae touch its alveolar processes instead of the horizontal ridges.

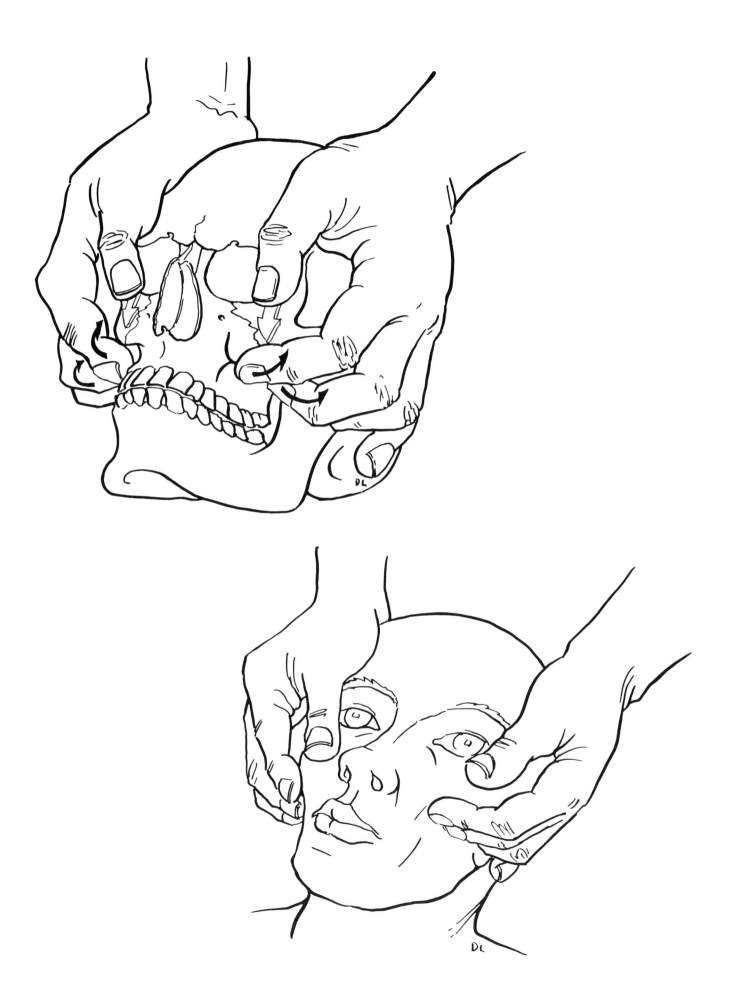

# UNILATERAL RELEASE OF THE MAXILLA

### Objective

To restore functional freedom to the maxilla during external and internal rotation.

### Position of the patient

Supine, comfortable and relaxed.

### Position of the practitioner

Seated at the patient's head, on the side opposite the lesion, the table adjusted to a convenient height.

### Points of contact

Cephalic hand: the clamp of the thumb and index finger spans the frontal bone, without making contact. The index finger and thumb are placed on the greater wings of the sphenoid.

Caudal hand: the intrabuccal index finger is placed on the maxilla beneath its zygomatic process.

### Movement

Direct correction of lesion in internal rotation: during the expansion phase, the intrabuccal index finger rolls caudally and externally around its longitudinal axis (without losing its contact), while the cephalic hand draws the sphenoid along in external rotation (flexion).

This maneuver is reversed, of course, for correction of a lesion in external rotation.

### Comment

It is imperative that the contact beneath the zygomatic process be intrabuccal. Making the same contact externally is part of an entirely different technique, in which the practitioner performs a lifting, rather than a rolling, of the bone, using the zygomatic process as a lever.

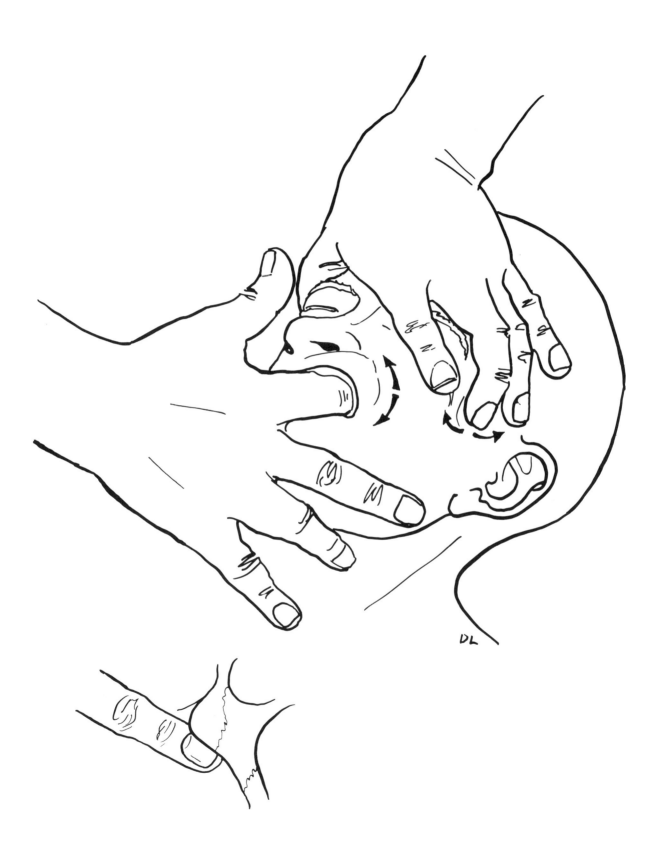

# BILATERAL RELEASE OF THE MAXILLAE

**Objective**

To restore functional freedom to both maxillae during external and internal rotation.

**Position of the patient**

Supine, comfortable and relaxed.

**Position of the practitioner**

Seated at the patient's head, forearms resting on the treatment table which has been adjusted to a convenient height.

**Points of contact**

The two hands are placed on either side of the patient's head. The thumbs rest on the zygomae. The index fingers (and in some cases, depending on the difference in size between the practitioner's hands and the subject's cranium, other fingers) are hooked under the palatine processes of the maxillae.

**Movement**

During the expansion phase of cranial motion, the thumbs follow the physiological movement of the zygomae. At the same time, the fingers hooked under the palatine processes of the maxillae begin moving apart horizontally.

During the relaxation phase, the practitioner terminates this maneuver, allowing a return to the neutral position.

This cycle is repeated until a release is perceived.

**Comment**

Because of the levers, the practitioner's action is very powerful; a measure of restraint is required.

The condition of the patient's gums or the presence of dental plates in the patient's mouth may prevent use of this technique.

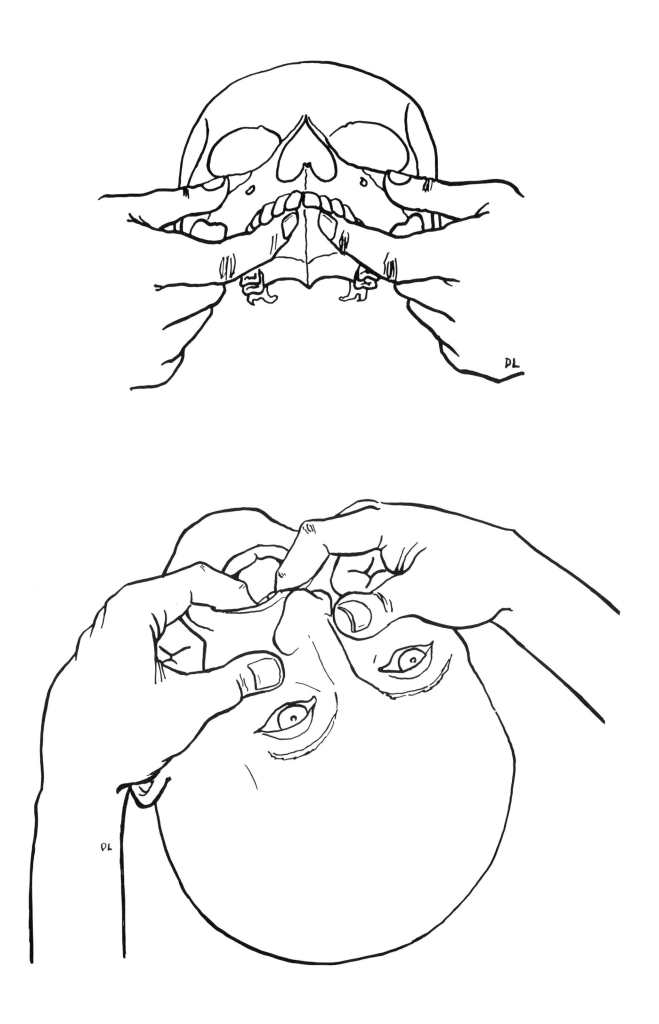

# MAXILLOETHMOID TECHNIQUE

### Objective

To restore harmony to the functional relationship between the maxilla and ethmoid bones. This technique plays an essential part in the ventilation of the sinuses.

### Position of the patient

Supine, comfortable and relaxed.

### Position of the practitioner

Seated at the patient's head, on the side opposite the lesion, the treatment table adjusted to a convenient height.

### Points of contact

The cephalic hand simultaneously controls the sphenoid and the frontal. The clamp of the thumb and index finger spans the frontal bone: the thumb touches the greater wing of the sphenoid with the interphalangeal articulation, and the external orbital process of the frontal with the pad of the terminal phalanx. On the opposite side, the middle and index fingers are placed on the corresponding points.

The caudal hand immobilizes the maxilla as follows:

— intrabuccal middle finger beneath the zygomatic process;

— index finger at the frontal process of the maxilla.

In an acceptable variation for the caudal hand, the index finger replaces the intrabuccal middle finger, and the thumb replaces the index finger at the frontal process.

### Movement

Only the cephalic hand is active; it repositions the ethmoid, through the frontal and sphenoid bones, on the maxilla (which is secured by the caudal hand).

During the expansion phase, the cephalic hand draws the frontal and sphenoid in flexion, in search of the articular balance with the maxilla through the ethmoid. When this point of balanced tension is found, it is held until a release is perceived.

### Comment

Because of the relative fragility of the ethmoid, this indirect technique requires a very light touch, without strong pressure.

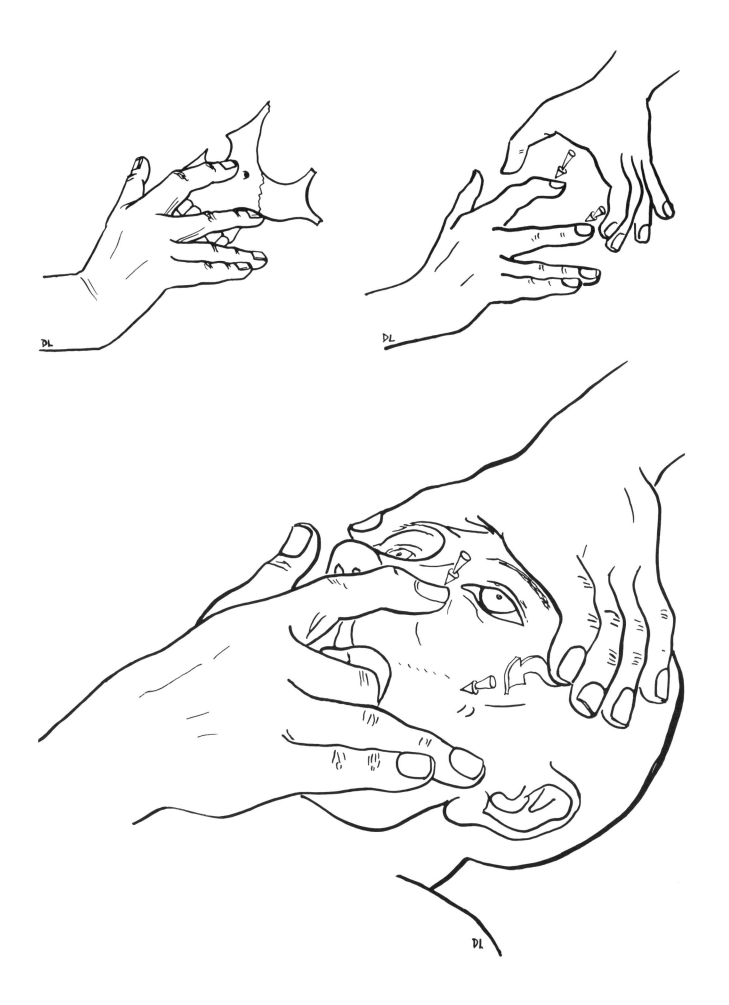

# MAXILLOPALATINE TECHNIQUE

**Objective**

To disengage the bevel of the maxillopalatine articulation.

**Position of the patient**

Supine, comfortable and relaxed.

**Position of the practitioner**

Seated at the patient's head, on the side opposite the lesion, the table adjusted to a convenient height.

**Points of contact**

The cephalic hand controls the sphenoid. The clamp of the thumb and index finger spans the frontal without making contact. The index finger and thumb are placed on the greater wings of the sphenoid.

On the caudal hand, the index finger is placed under the palatine process of the maxilla, with the phalanx at the superior incisor. If a stronger action is desired, the middle finger can be placed under the palatine process and its action reinforced by positioning the index finger under the zygomatic process.

**Movement**

During the expansion phase the practitioner, with the caudal hand, lowers the palatine process of the maxilla (bevelled superiorly), by externally rotating this bone.

At the same time, the sphenoid is drawn into extension by the cephalic hand, which thereby brings the maxillary process of the palatine (bevelled inferiorly) in a cephalic direction. This is held until a release is perceived. Thereafter, both the maxilla and the palatine (via the sphenoid) are drawn into external rotation during the next expansion phase of the cranial mechanism.

**Comment**

This technique is performed during the expansion phase of cranial motion, even though the sphenoid is drawn into extension, because the affected sutures have been shown to be most open during this phase.

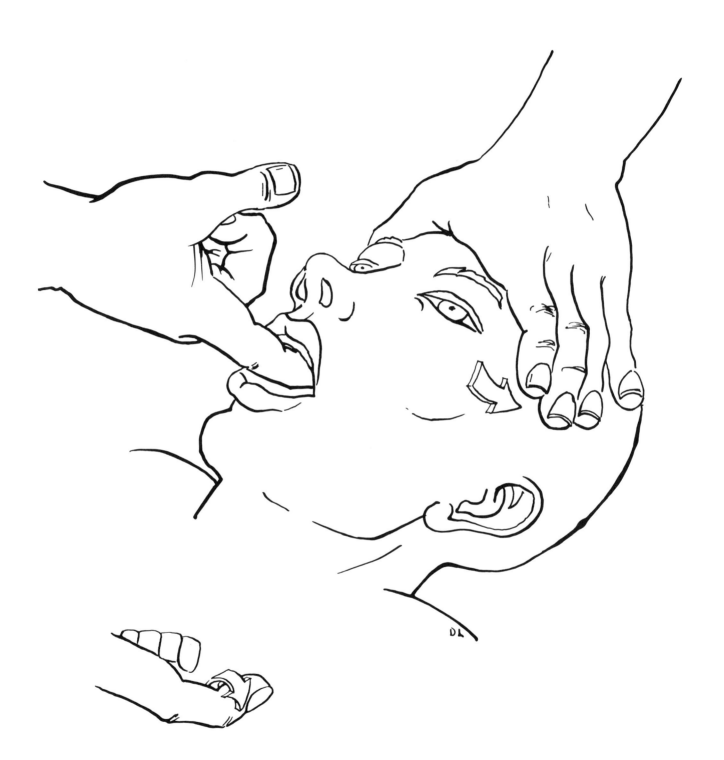

# MAXILLONASAL TECHNIQUE

**Objective**

To restore functional freedom to the articulation between the maxilla and nasal bones.

**Position of the patient**

Supine, comfortable and relaxed.

**Position of the practitioner**

Seated at the patient's head, the treatment table adjusted to a convenient height.

**Points of contact**

The pads of thumb and index finger on the cephalic hand come together, forming a V-shaped notch and covering the two nasal bones.

The intrabuccal index finger of the caudal hand is lodged under the zygomatic process on the lateral surface of the affected maxilla.

**Movement**

The cephalic hand immobilizes the nasal bones in external rotation.

The intrabuccal index finger rolls around its longitudinal axis, initiating external rotation during the expansion phase, then internal rotation during the relaxation phase, in search of the articular balance. This is held until a release is perceived.

**Comment**

To obtain articular freedom, it is sometimes necessary to exert a cephalad traction on the nasal bones.

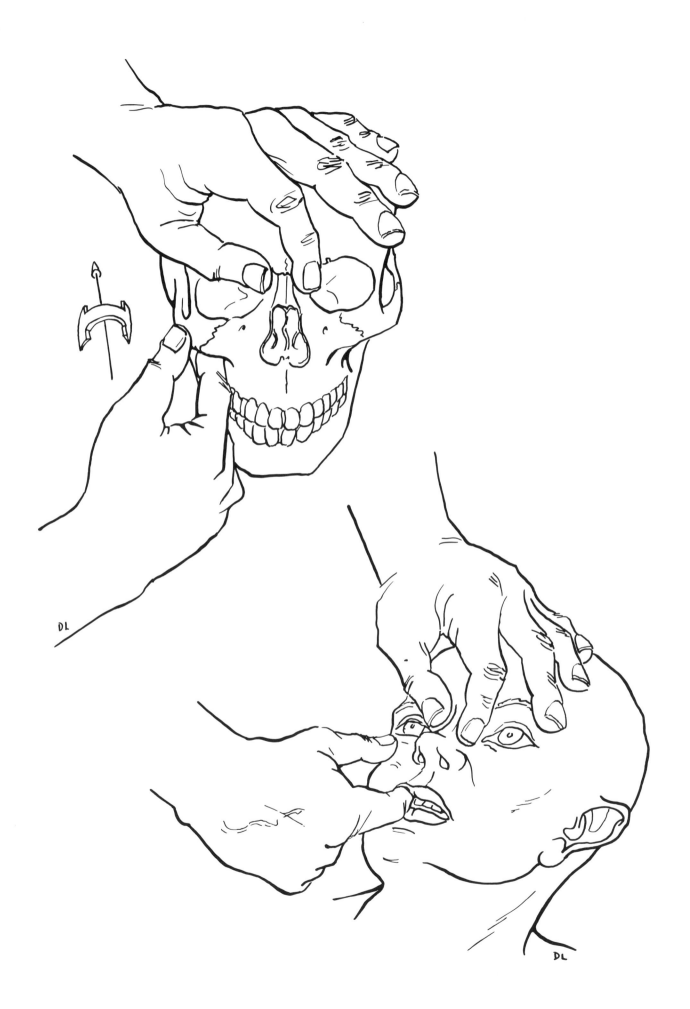

# INTERMAXILLARY TECHNIQUE

**Objective**

To restore functional freedom between the two maxillae.

**Position of the patient**

Supine, comfortable and relaxed.

**Position of the practitioner**

Seated at one side of the patient's head, the treatment table adjusted to a convenient height.

**Points of contact**

The palm of the cephalic hand is positioned on the frontal bone. Thumb and index finger are on the zygomae beneath their orbital border.

On the caudal hand, the palmar sides of the terminal phalanges of index finger and middle finger are placed under the palatine process of the right and left maxillae.

**Movement**

During the expansion phase of the cranial mechanism, the cephalic hand, using its palm, draws the frontal in flexion while the thumb and index finger accentuate the external rotation of the zygomae caudally and laterally.

Simultaneously, the intraoral index and middle fingers of the caudal hand draw apart from each other, while pushing the palatine processes slightly toward the back of the mouth.

**Comment**

Because the mouth is a slippery area, the practitioner must make the intraoral contacts very carefully and not release them through the entire course of the maneuver.

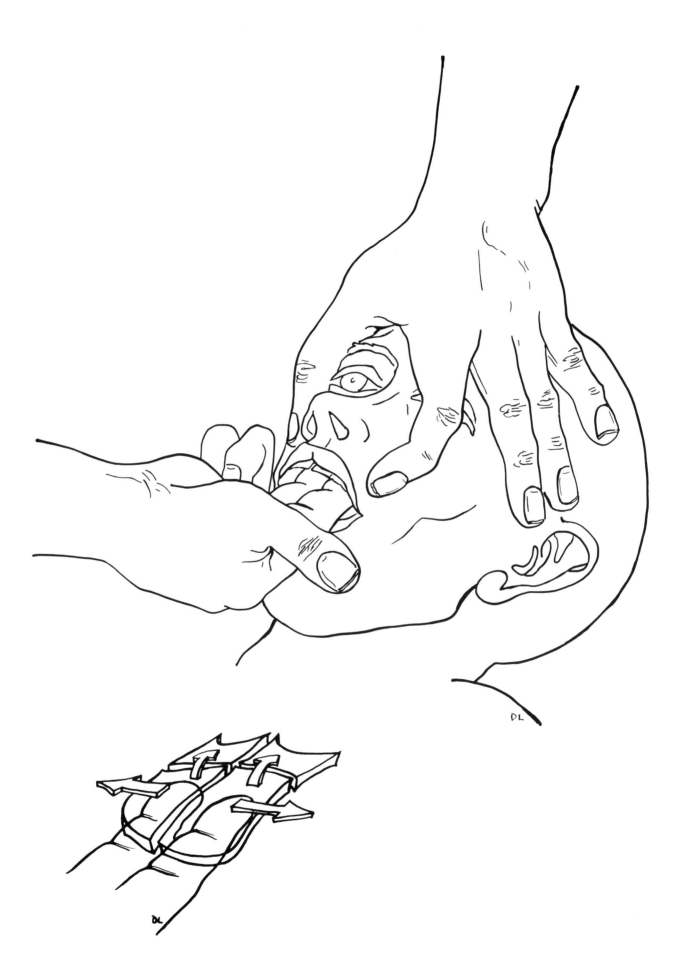

# REPOSITIONING OF THE MAXILLA

### Objective

To restore the functional relationship of the maxilla with the neighboring bones after trauma.

### Position of the patient

Supine, comfortable and relaxed.

### Position of the practitioner

Seated at the patient's head, on the side of the lesion, the treatment table adjusted to a convenient height.

### Points of contact

The thenar eminence of the cephalic hand is placed on that part of the frontal which is just cephalad to the lesion; the pad of the terminal phalanx of the thumb is on the superior frontal process of the injured maxilla; and the other fingers are spread over the frontal.

The caudal hand grasps the maxilla above the teeth with the thumb and index finger. The thumb is placed on the buccal surface of the bone, behind the canine eminence; and the index finger is positioned on the lingual surface, under the palatine process.

### Movement

During the expansion phase, the cephalic hand encourages the frontal in flexion; during the expansion phase, in extension.

Simultaneously, the thumb on the frontal process draws the latter in a coronal (external rotation) and then sagittal (internal rotation) plane.

The caudal hand moves the maxilla into a position of balanced tension around the axis of the frontal process. This should be maintained until a release is perceived. In most cases there will be a different position for each phase of the cranial rhythm.

### Comment

This is a particularly effective manipulation which requires a light touch on the part of the practitioner.

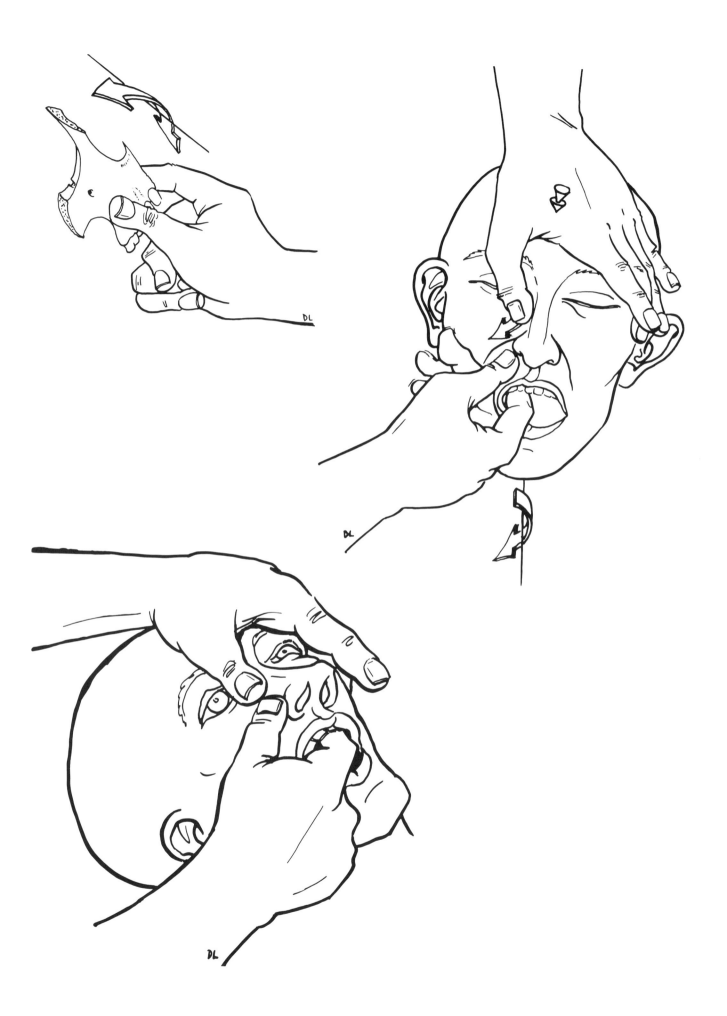

# DRAINAGE OF THE MAXILLARY SINUS

**Objective**

To increase the ventilation of the maxillary sinus. This technique will cause the drainage of purulent secretions which have been abnormally held there.

**Position of the patient**

Supine, comfortable and relaxed.

**Position of the practitioner**

Seated at the patient's head, on the side opposite the lesion, the treatment table adjusted to a convenient height.

**Points of contact**

The cephalic hand mobilizes the sphenoid and frontal with the clamp of the thumb and index finger. The thumb touches the greater wing of the sphenoid and the external orbital process of the frontal bone on the side opposite the lesion, while the index and middle fingers are placed on the corresponding points on the side of the lesion.

The caudal hand controls the facial bones as follows:

—thumb on the superior frontal process of the maxilla;

—index finger on the zygoma;

—middle finger intrabuccal under the zygomatic process of the maxilla;

—little finger intraoral along the intermaxillary suture.

**Movement**

The cephalic hand accentuates the flexion motion of the frontal bone and of the sphenoid during the expansion phase. At the same time, the other hand draws the facial bones in external rotation: the middle finger revolves around its longitudinal axis; the index finger rolls the zygoma caudally and laterally; the little finger moves the intermaxillary suture cephalad and anteriorly. This causes better ventilation of the sinus.

Both hands perform the opposite movement during the relaxation phase.

This promotes drainage of the maxillary sinus. To be effective this process must be continued until a release is perceived, usually in two to three minutes.

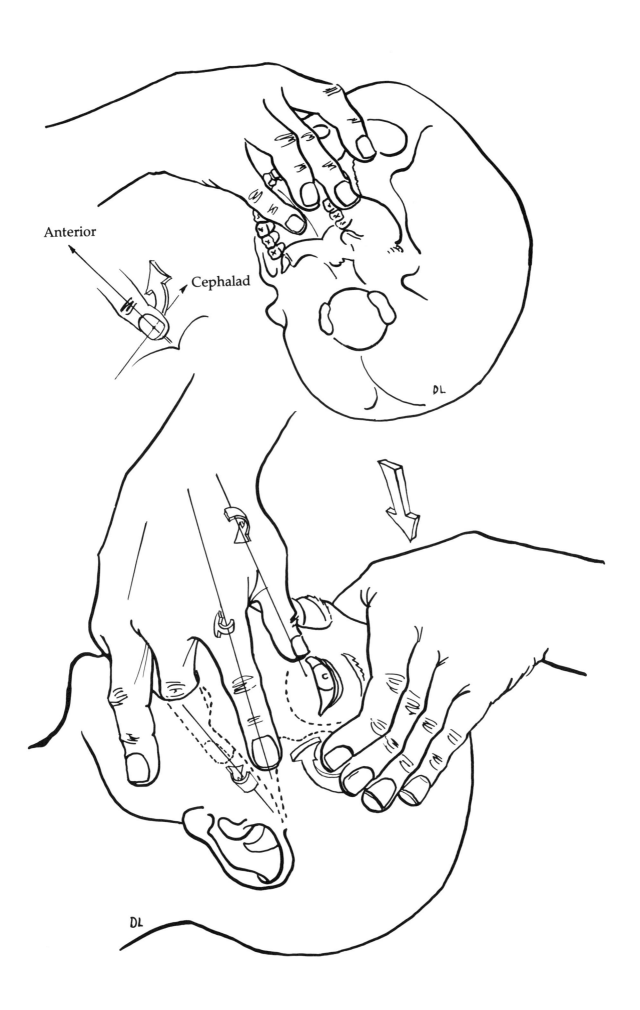

Anterior

Cephalad

# UNILATERAL RELEASE OF THE ETHMOID

## FACIAL APPROACH

**Objective**

To unilaterally free the physiological motion of the ethmoid within the general motion of the cranium.

**Position of the patient**

Supine, comfortable and relaxed.

**Position of the practitioner**

Seated at the patient's head, on the side opposite the lesion.

**Points of contact**

The cephalic hand spans the frontal bone with the clamp of the thumb and index finger. The terminal phalanges of the thumb and index finger are placed behind the two external orbital processes.

On the side of the lesion, the ring finger of the caudal hand is placed on the zygoma; the middle finger on the anterolateral surface of the maxilla; and the index finger on the frontal process of the maxilla.

**Movement**

During the expansion phase of cranial motion, the cephalic hand accentuates the flexion of the frontal, with the palm lowering the glabella and moving back the metopic suture toward the vertex. The thumb and index finger push the external orbital processes anteriorly and caudally.

The caudal hand draws the facial bones in external rotation. The ring finger moves the zygoma caudally and laterally, and the middle and index fingers move the maxilla. This leads to the point of balanced tension which is maintained until a release is perceived.

**Comment**

Because the ethmoid cannot be touched directly, this technique, to be effective, requires scrupulous attention to the correct points of contact.

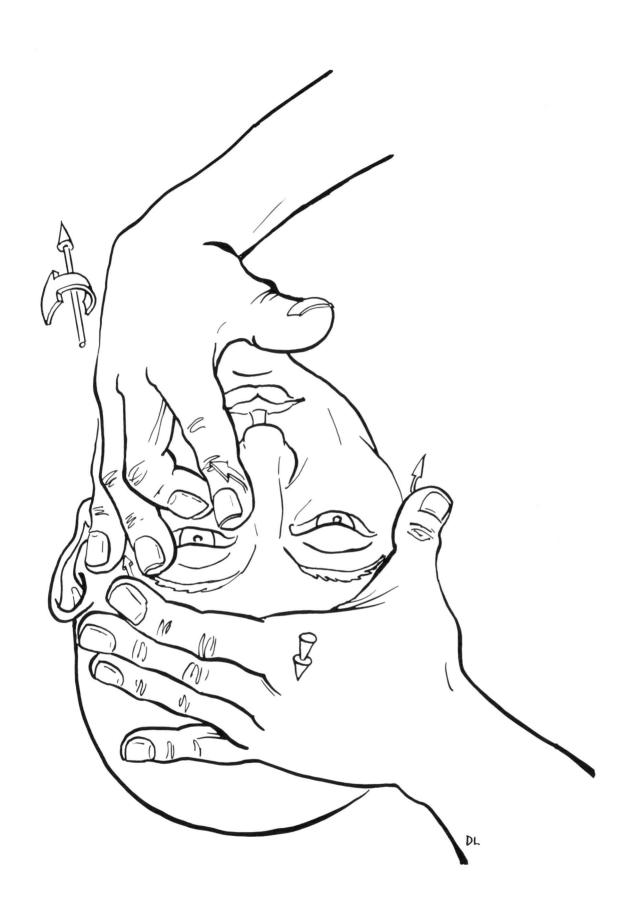

# RELEASE OF THE ETHMOID PERPENDICULAR PLATE

**Objective**

To restore freedom of motion to the perpendicular plate of the ethmoid in relation to the neighboring bones.

**Position of the patient**

Supine, comfortable and relaxed.

**Position of the practitioner**

Seated beside the table at the patient's head.

**Points of contact**

The cephalic hand holds the sphenoid and the frontal in position with the clamp of the thumb and index finger. The thumb touches the greater wing of the sphenoid and the external orbital process of the frontal. On the other side, the index and middle fingers are placed on the corresponding points.

The caudal hand is held symmetrically to the other hand and controls the two superior maxillae.

**Movement**

During the expansion phase of cranial motion, the cephalic hand draws the sphenoid and the frontal in flexion (the greater wings and orbital processes moved caudally and anteriorly), while lowering the metopic sutures. At the same time, the caudal hand initiates the external rotation of the two maxillae. This leads to a point of balanced tension which is maintained until a release is perceived.

**Comment**

The action of both hands must be perfectly coordinated. To be effective, any indirect maneuver such as this requires precise hand movements.

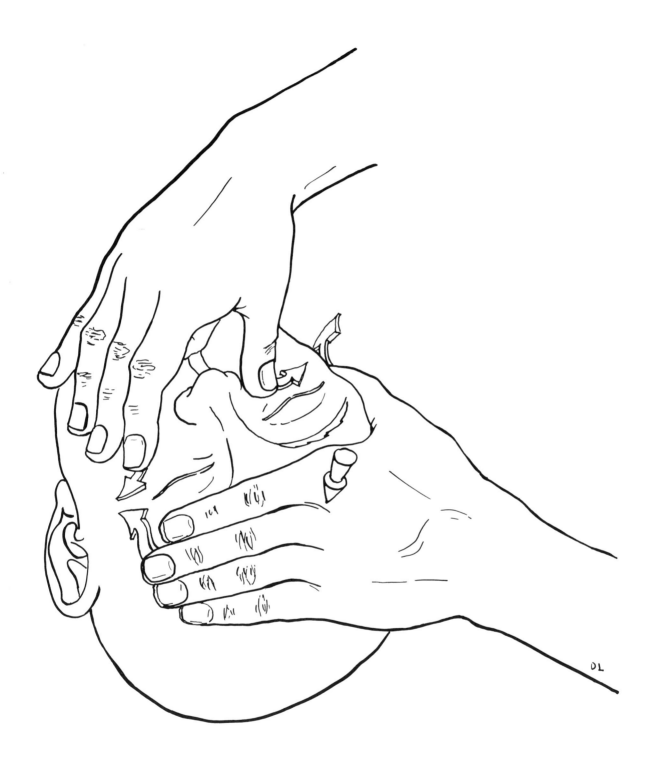

# RELEASE OF THE CRIBIFORM PLATE

## Objective

To free the cribiform plate, within the general motion of the cranium, at the ethmoidal notch of the frontal.

## Position of the patient

Supine, comfortable and relaxed.

## Position of the practitioner

Seated at the patient's head, to one side of the treatment table.

## Points of contact

On the cephalic hand, the clamp of the thumb and index finger spans the frontal. The terminal phalanges of thumb and index finger are placed behind the two external orbital processes of the bone.

On the caudal hand, the thumb and ring finger are both placed on the anterolateral surfaces of the maxillae. The index and middle fingers are positioned on the frontal processes of these same bones.

## Movement

1st phase:  the cephalic hand compresses the frontal during the relaxation phase. This reduces the ethmoidal notch of the frontal and releases the fixation.

2nd phase:  during the expansion phase, while the caudal hand maintains both maxillae in external rotation, the cephalic hand lifts the frontal in flexion. This is continued until a release is perceived.

## Comment

It is possible for the practitioner to make the effect of this technique unilateral. To this end, the practitioner places the index finger of the caudal hand in the mouth under the zygomatic process of the maxilla on the side of the lesion. The thumb may be placed on the frontal process of the same bone. The technique then follows the movement described above.

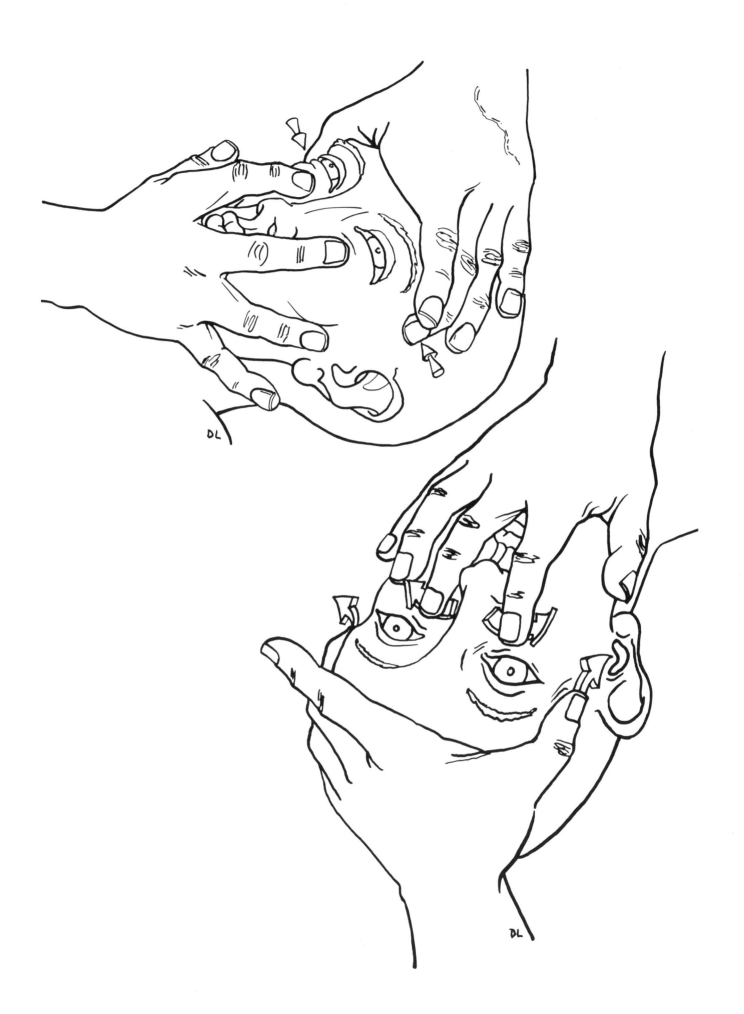

# RELEASE OF THE ETHMOID LATERAL MASSES

## Objective

To restore the ventilation function to the lateral masses of the ethmoid by releasing the neighboring bones.

## Position of the patient

Sitting on the edge of the treatment table, which has been adjusted to a convenient height.

## Position of the practitioner

Standing at one side of, and facing the patient.

## Points of contact

The cephalic hand grasps the frontal with the clamp of the thumb and index finger, which are placed behind the external orbital processes.

The index finger of the caudal hand is placed on the cruciate suture of the palate.

## Movement

After a deep inhalation the patient holds his or her breath in and bends the head forward. The palate leans on the practitioner's index finger. The practitioner's cephalic hand draws the frontal bone in external rotation.

This maneuver must be repeated until a release is perceived.

## Comment

This technique may be performed on a supine patient. In that case, the intraoral index finger of the practitioner, instead of merely supporting the palate, becomes active at the same time as the cephalic hand.

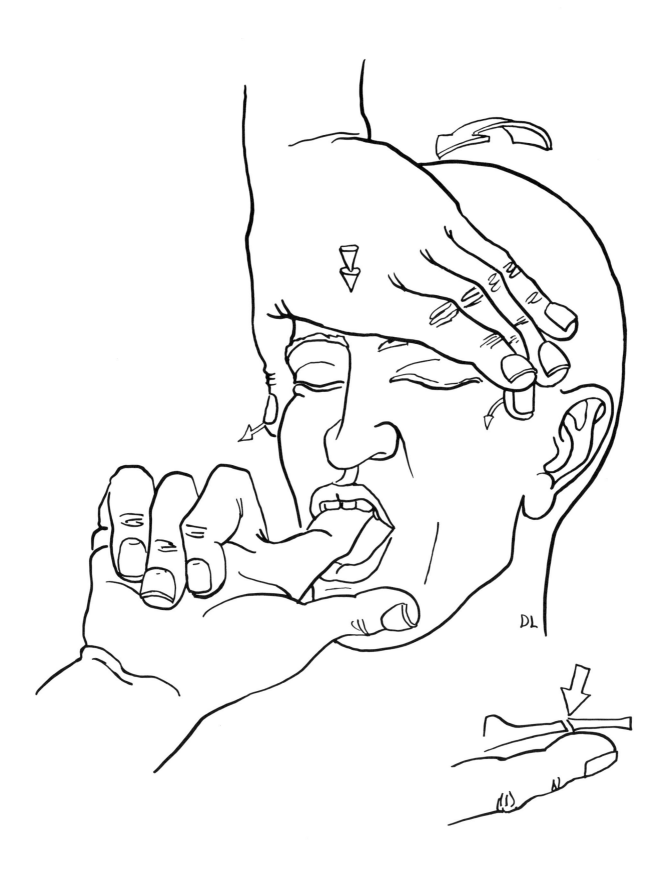

# DRAINAGE OF THE ETHMOIDAL SINUS

**Objective**

To induce a pumping action, causing the release and discharge of purulent secretions stagnating in the ethmoidal sinus.

**Position of the patient**

Supine, comfortable and relaxed.

**Position of the practitioner**

Seated and facing the patient's head, on the side opposite the lesion.

**Points of contact**

On the cephalic hand, the palm clasps the frontal; the thumb is behind the external orbital process of the bone; and the other fingers are spread out on the facial bones on the side of the lesion. The little and ring fingers secure the zygoma, and the maxilla is held steady by the middle finger placed on the anterolateral surface. The index finger is positioned on the frontal process of the maxilla.

The index finger of the caudal hand is placed on the cruciate suture of the palate.

**Movement**

During the expansion phase, the cephalic hand draws the frontal, the zygoma and the maxilla in external rotation, while the intrabuccal index finger presses the palate cephalad and anteriorly toward the root of the nose. The physiological movement is thus clearly amplified.

Both hands perform the opposite movement during the relaxation phase.

These two phases must be repeated several times until a release is perceived.

**Comment**

Ethmoidal sinus congestion is often caused by a problem somewhere else. Once the ventilation of the sinus is achieved, the practitioner must release the primary, causal lesion.

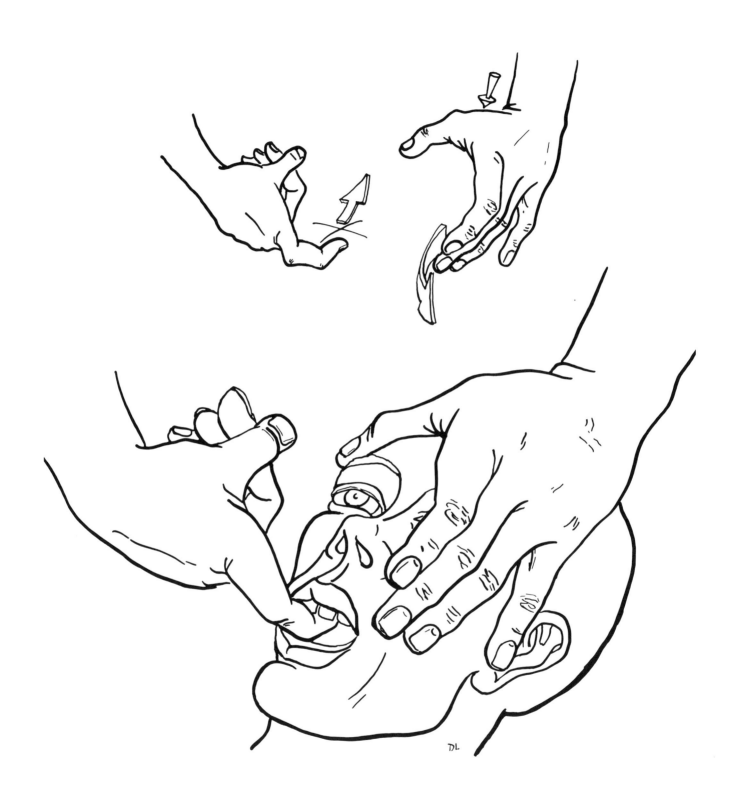

# RELEASE OF THE ZYGOMA

## FIRST TECHNIQUE

**Objective**

To reestablish the physiological and functional freedom of the zygoma during external and internal rotation.

**Position of the patient**

Supine, comfortable and relaxed.

**Position of the practitioner**

Seated at the patient's head, forearms resting on the treatment table which has been adjusted to a convenient height. The practitioner holds the patient's head in his or her hands.

**Points of contact**

The index fingers of the hands touch the zygomae just under the orbital border, while the distal phalanges of the middle fingers rest on the inferior border of the zygomae.

**Movement**

During the expansion phase, the palms of the hands follow the external rotation motion of the bones they are covering. At the same time, the index fingers draw along the external rotation of the orbital border of the zygomae, an action which is reinforced by the pressure of the middle fingers caudally and medially.

During the relaxation phase, the fingers perform the movements in reverse.

When a point of balanced tension is found, it is maintained until a release is perceived.

NOTE: This bilateral maneuver may be performed on one side only, as illustrated on the opposite page. The other hand on the frontal helps with the release of the frontozygomatic bone.

**Comment**

This harmonious technique is insufficient to deal with an impaction of the zygoma. In that case, use the technique described on page 210.

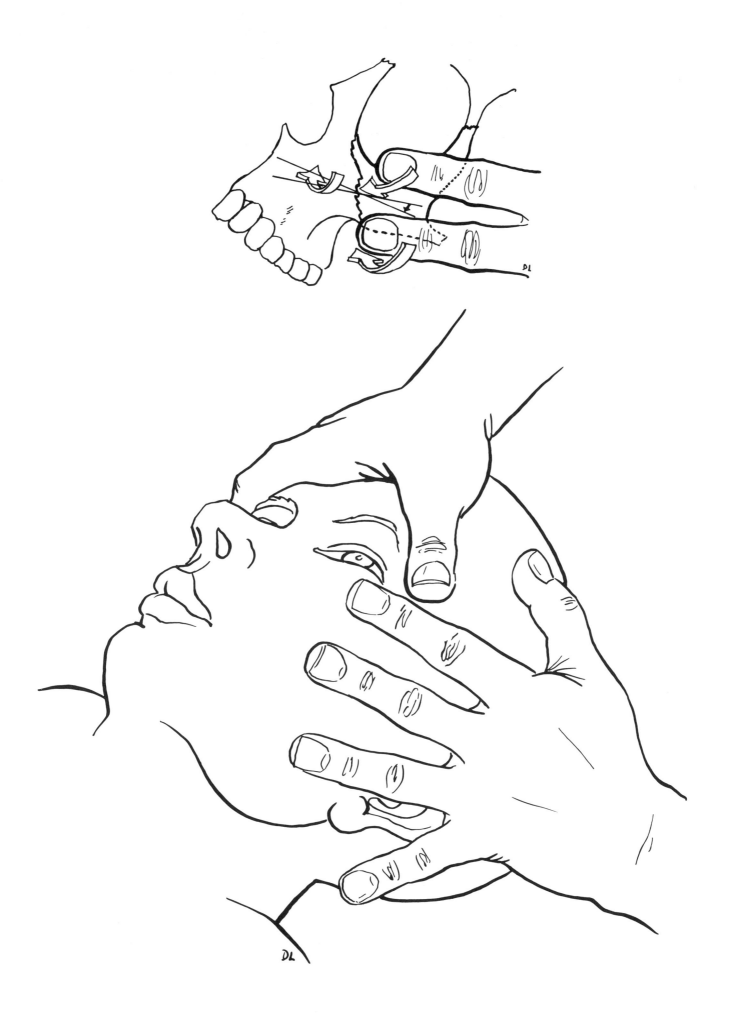

# RELEASE OF THE ZYGOMA

## SECOND TECHNIQUE

### Objective

To reestablish the physiological motion of the zygoma during both phases of the cranial mechanism.

### Position of the patient

Supine, comfortable and relaxed.

### Position of the practitioner

Seated at the patient's head, on the side of the lesion, the table adjusted to a convenient height.

### Points of contact

The palm of the cephalic hand cups the frontal; the index finger is placed behind the opposite external orbital process; the thenar eminence is positioned on the frontal eminence on the side of the lesion; and the pad of the terminal phalanx of the thumb touches the superior border of the zygoma.

The index finger of the caudal hand is intrabuccal, placed supine under the inferior border of the lesioned zygoma.

### Movement

During the expansion phase, the thumb of the cephalic hand draws the superior border of the zygoma laterally and caudally (in external rotation), while the intrabuccal index finger accentuates this movement.

During the relaxation phase, the same fingers perform the opposite movement (internal rotation).

When a point of balanced tension is found, it is maintained until a release is perceived.

### Comment

This technique, stronger than the one on page 208 and gentler than that on page 212, has the disadvantage of requiring pressure on sensitive points.

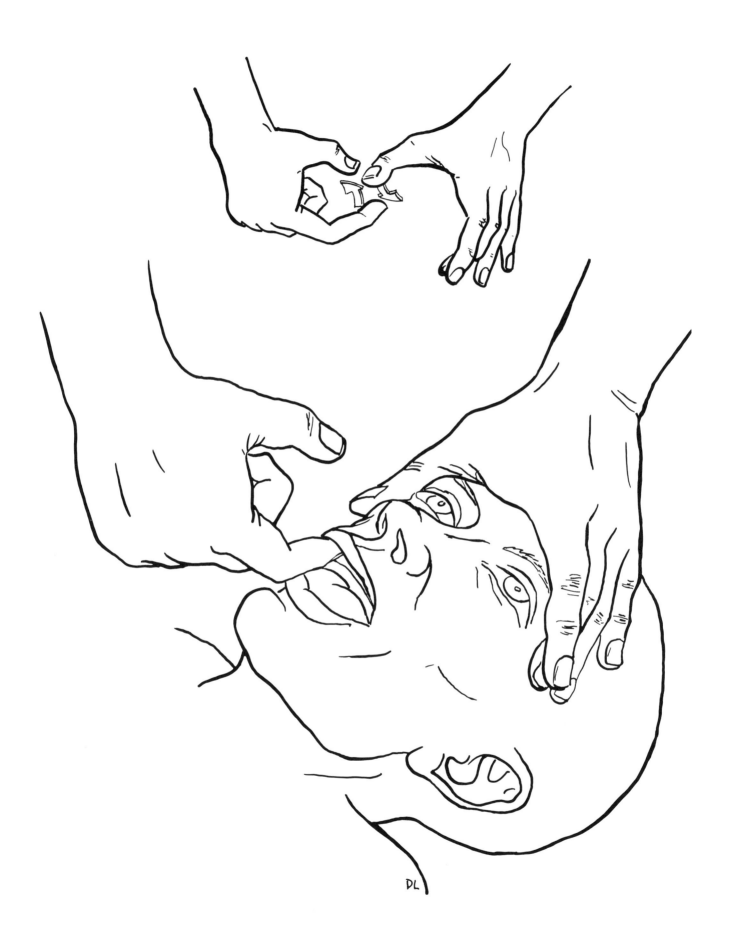

# BALANCING OF THE ZYGOMA

### Objective

To restore the functional relationship of the zygoma with the neighboring bones within the motion of the cranial mechanism.

### Position of the patient

Supine, comfortable and relaxed.

### Position of the practitioner

Seated at the patient's head, on the side of the lesion.

### Points of contact

The cephalic hand cups the cranial vault. The thumb is placed perpendicular to the zygomatic process of the temporal.

The caudal hand grasps the zygoma between the thumb and index finger, with the thumb on the cheek and the index finger intrabuccal.

### Movement

During the expansion phase of cranial motion, the thumb of the cephalic hand accentuates the external rotation of the temporal (disengagement of the temporozygomatic articulation). At the same time, the caudal hand repositions the zygoma in external rotation.

The practitioner should regard the relaxation phase as a neutral phase during which he or she does nothing but follow along with the motion.

This process is repeated until a release is perceived.

### Comment

The intrabuccal index finger presses on the mucous membrane which lines the internal surface of the zygoma. Because this membrane is generally very sensitive, it is important that the pressure be gentle.

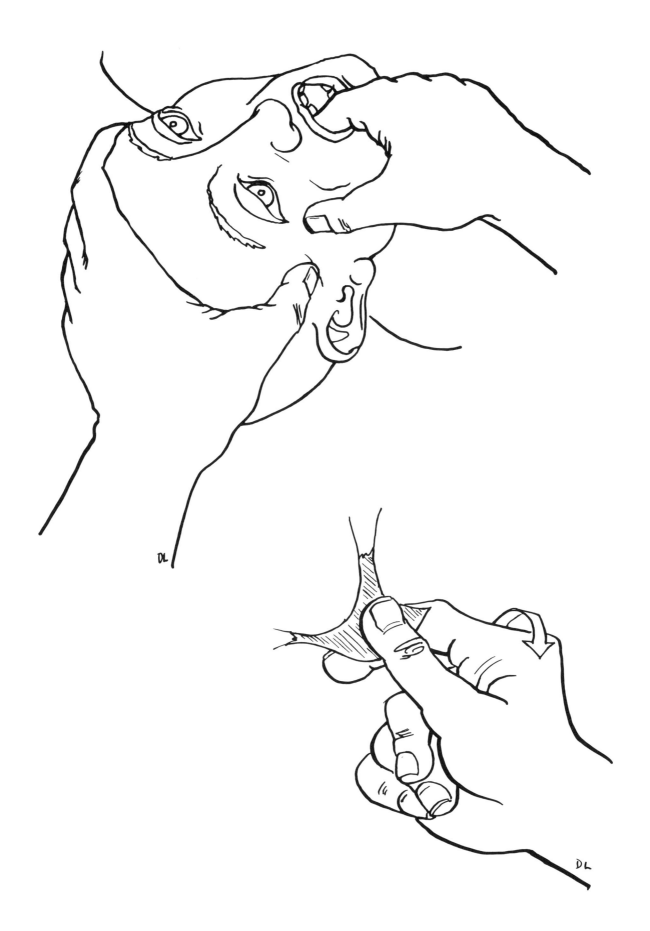

# ZYGOMATIC MAXILLA RELEASE

### Objective

To normalize the mobility of the zygomatic-maxillary articulation, the impaction of which, usually traumatic, occurs frequently.

### Position of the patient

Supine, comfortable and relaxed.

### Position of the practitioner

Seated at the patient's head, on the side of the lesion.

### Points of contact

The cephalic hand clasps the zygoma between the thumb, which is placed on the orbital border, and the index finger, placed on the inferior border of the bone.

The index finger of the caudal hand is positioned intrabuccally under the zygomatic process of the maxilla.

If necessary, the action of this finger may be reinforced by that of the thumb, which is placed on the external surface of the cheek behind the canine tuberosity.

### Movement

With the intrabuccal index finger used as a base, the other hand initiates the external rotation of the zygoma (caudally and laterally) during the expansion phase, and its internal rotation during the relaxation phase. When a point of balanced tension is found, it is maintained until a release is perceived.

### Comment

When the release of the zygomatic-maxillary articulation has been obtained, the practitioner must make sure that the zygoma's motion is perfectly integrated within the general cranial motion.

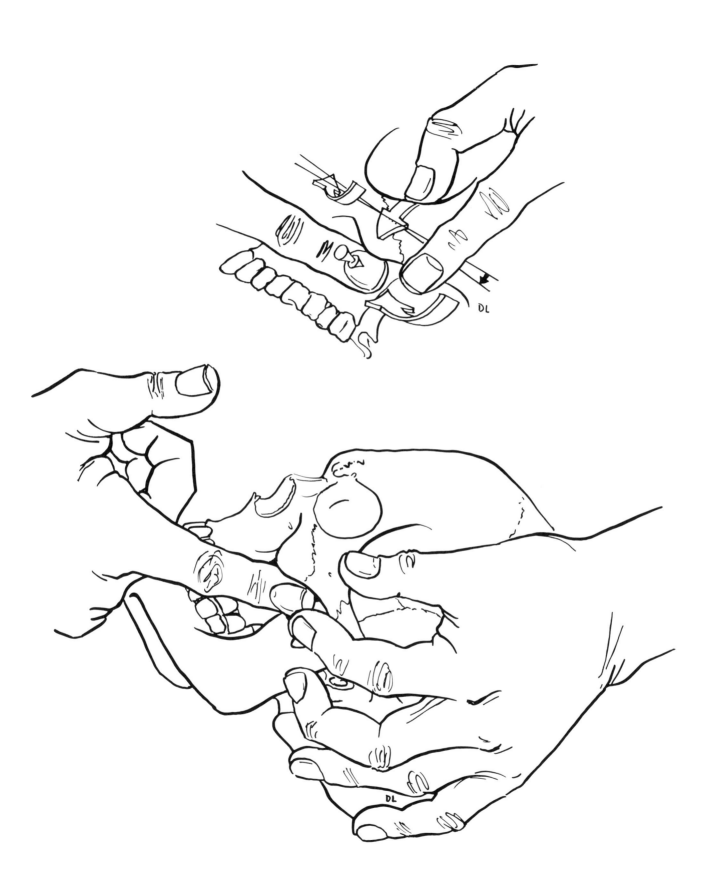

# PTERYGOPALATINE RELEASE

**Objective**

To restore functional freedom between the pyramidal process of the palatine bone and the pterygoid process of the sphenoid.

**Position of the patient**

Supine, comfortable and relaxed.

**Position of the practitioner**

Seated at the patient's head, on the side of the lesion.

**Points of contact**

On the cephalic hand, the clamp of the thumb and index finger cups the frontal bone; these fingers are positioned on the greater wings of the sphenoid.

The pad on the index finger of the caudal hand touches the palatine bone near the medial line. The middle joint takes a firm base on the first upper molar.

**Movement**

From its base on the first upper molar, and without losing contact with the horizontal process of the palatine, the practitioner turns the pad of the intraoral index finger toward the cheek and keeps it there. He or she then draws the bone along anterolaterally, disengaging it from the pterygoid process.

During the expansion phase, the practitioner moves the sphenoid on its transverse and anteroposterior axes in search of the balance point. When this is found, it is held until a release is perceived.

**Comment**

The difficulty of this technique proceeds from the thinness of the horizontal process of the palatine, which requires uninterrupted contact with the pad of the index finger throughout the maneuver.

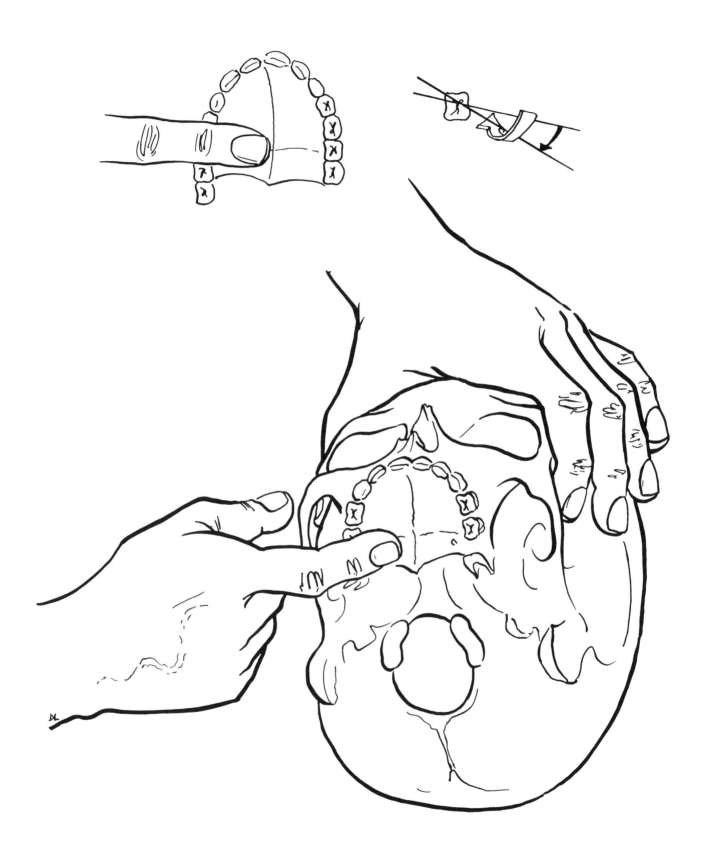

# INTERPALATINE RELEASE

**Objective**

To restore functional freedom between the two horizontal processes of the palatine bones.

**Position of the patient**

Supine, comfortable and relaxed.

**Position of the practitioner**

Facing the patient's head.

**Points of contact**

The thumb and index finger clamp of the cephalic hand cups the frontal, with the terminal phalanges placed on the greater wings of the sphenoid.

The pad on the index finger of the caudal hand touches the palatine on the side of the lesion near the medial line. The phalanx takes a firm hold on the first upper molar. The middle finger, leaning against the index finger, touches the horizontal process of the other palatine.

**Movement**

From its base on the first molar, and without losing the contacts with the palate, the practitioner turns the pad of the index finger toward the corresponding cheek, and at the same time turns the middle finger (distal side) toward the other cheek. The fingers are kept in this position.

During the expansion phase, the practitioner moves the sphenoid on its transverse and anteroposterior axes in search of the balance point. When this is found, it is held until a release is perceived.

**Comment**

The difficulty of this technique proceeds from the thinness of the horizontal process of the palatine, which requires uninterrupted contact with the pad of the index finger throughout the maneuver.

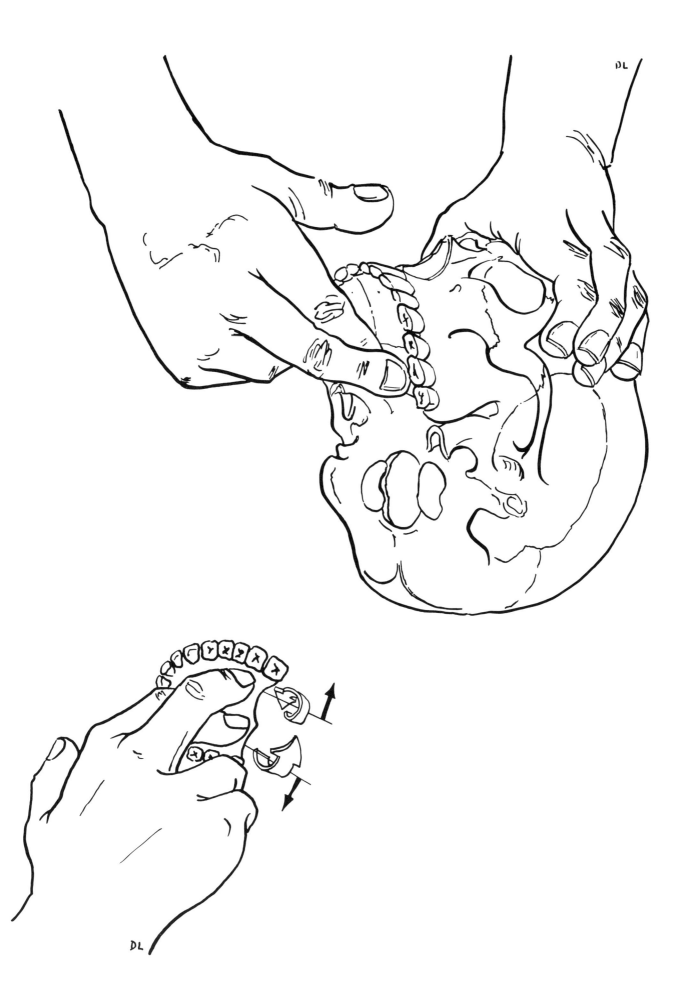

# REPOSITIONING OF THE VOMER

## Objective

To restore the functional relationship of the vomer between the palatine bones and the sphenoid.

## Position of the patient

Supine, comfortable and relaxed.

## Position of the practitioner

Seated and facing the patient's head, the treatment table adjusted to a convenient height.

## Points of contact

The cephalic hand controls the sphenoid. The clamp of the thumb and index finger cups the frontal without actually making contact. The terminal phalanges of the thumb and index finger are placed on the greater wings of the sphenoid.

The pad of the index finger of the caudal hand is placed under the cruciate suture of the palate.

## Movement

During the expansion phase, the cephalic hand draws the sphenoid along in flexion (greater wings caudad and anterior), while the intraoral index finger pulls the palate anteriorly toward the root of the nose.

During the relaxation phase, the sphenoidal hand performs this movement in reverse. At the same time, the intraoral index finger pushes the cruciate suture cephalad, toward the body of the sphenoid. These movements are repeated until a release is perceived.

## Comment

This technique bears a strong resemblance to the technique for drainage of the sphenoidal sinus (page 172). The two techniques, however, do have an operational difference. In the drainage of the sphenoidal sinus, the hands effect oppositional movements in order to bring about a discharge of secretions.

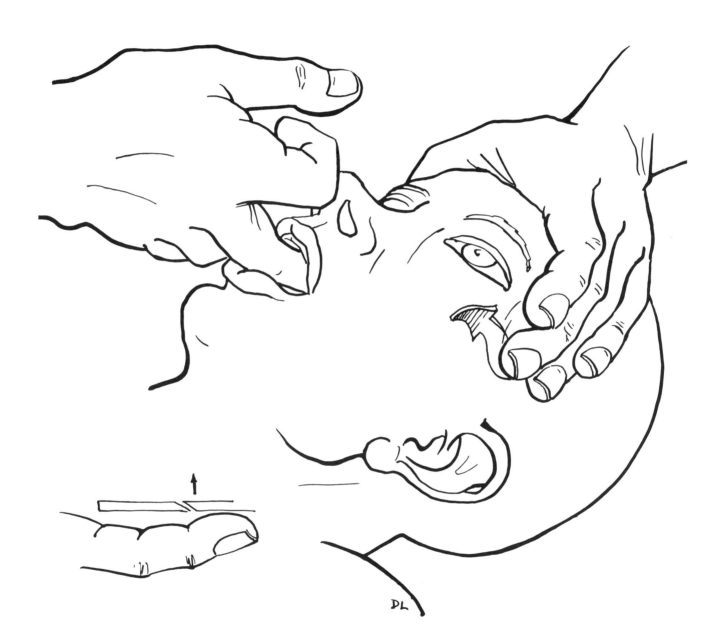

# STIMULATION OF THE SPHENOPALATINE GANGLION

**Objective**

To stimulate the sphenopalatine ganglion, which can increase cerebral circulation.

**Position of the patient**

Supine, comfortable and relaxed.

**Position of the practitioner**

Seated and facing the patient's head on the side opposite the ganglion to be stimulated, the treatment table adjusted to a convenient height.

**Points of contact**

The practitioner asks the patient to move his or her mandible to the side of the ganglion to be stimulated, both to facilitate the penetration of the practitioner's finger and to enlarge the fossa. The practitioner then inserts the index finger (or little finger, if it is long enough) of the caudal hand between the cheek and the alveolar border of the superior maxilla. The practitioner traces the latter to its end and proceeds along the pterygoid lamina. He or she penetrates the pterygopalatine fossa and encounters the resistant mass of tissues surrounding the ganglion. The pad of the finger is held there.

**Movement**

The practitioner asks the patient to turn his or her head toward the practitioner and bend it anteriorly, thus creating some pressure from the finger on the soft tissues in the pterygopalatine fossa and stimulating the ganglion. The practitioner may increase this effect by a slight vibration. This position is held until the tissues relax.

In an acceptable variation, this technique may be performed on a patient sitting on the edge of the treatment table and leaning on the practitioner's intrabuccal finger.

**Comment**

This technique provokes a number of reactions, the most common of which is watering of the eyes.

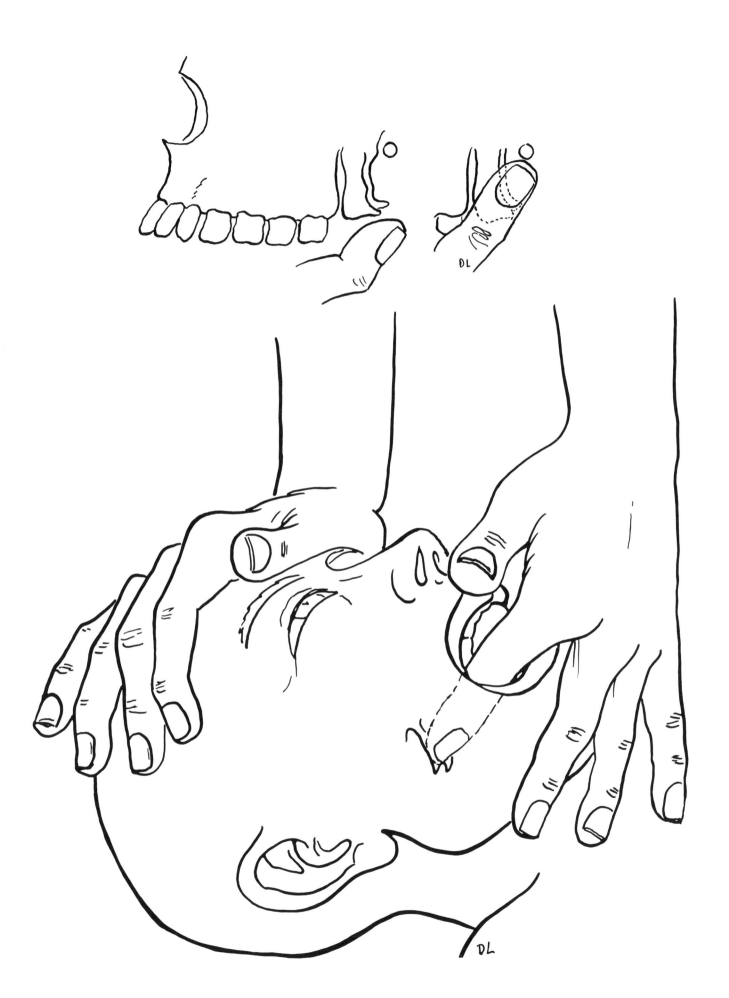

# NARROWING OF THE ORBIT

**Objective**

To restore proper dimension to the orbital cavity, i.e., narrowing it when it is too wide.

**Position of the patient**

Supine, comfortable and relaxed.

**Position of the practitioner**

Seated at the patient's head, on the side opposite the lesion.

**Points of contact**

The thumb of the cephalic hand is placed on the orbital margin of the frontal bone. The other fingers, which play no part in the maneuver, are spread out on the cranium.

The caudal hand controls the facial bones as follows:

—index finger in front of the frontozygomatic articulation;

—middle finger on the inferior border of the zygoma;

—thumb on the orbital margin of the superior maxilla.

**Movement**

During the relaxation phase, the frontal thumb pushes toward the center of the orbit. At the same time, the fingers of the caudal hand perform the following movements:

—index finger closes the frontozygomatic angle;

—middle finger accentuates the inversion (internal rotation) of the zygoma;

—thumb presses the inferior orbital margin toward the center of the eye.

During the expansion phase, the fingers gently resist the return to a neutral position. These movements are repeated until a release is perceived.

In one accepted variation of this technique, the practitioner sits on the side of the lesion and places the index finger of the cephalad hand on the orbital margin of the frontal bone, with the thumb on the frontozygomatic articulation. The thumb of the caudal hand is placed on the orbital margin of the maxilla.

**Comment**

This technique, which is easy to perform, nevertheless requires precise coordination of all the fingers.

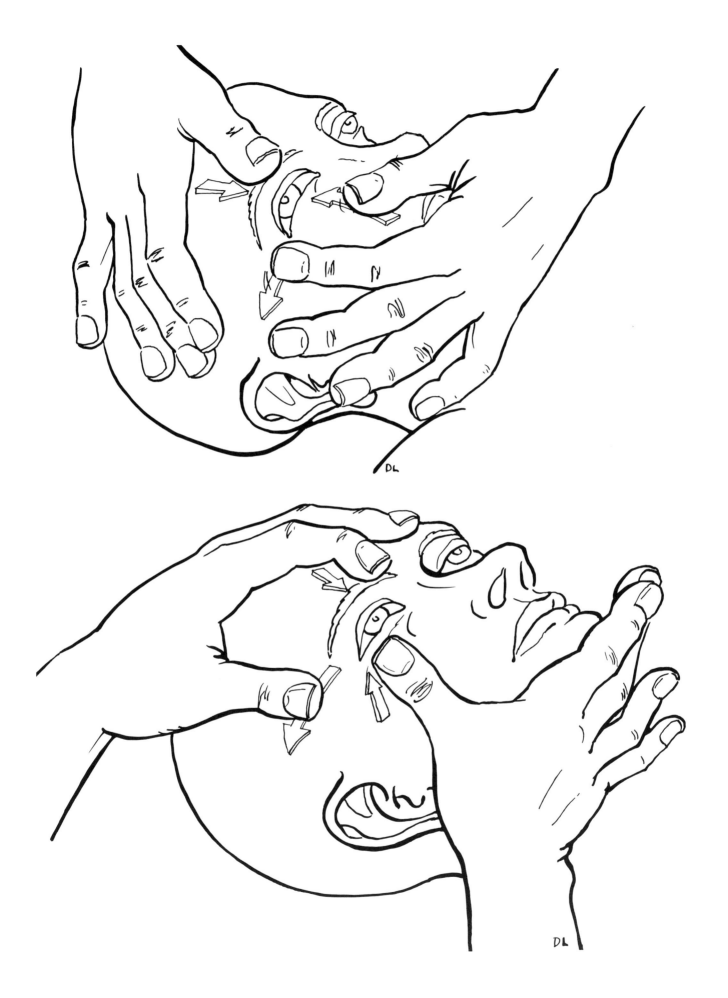

# WIDENING OF THE ORBIT

**Objective**

To restore proper dimension to the orbital cavity, i.e., enlarging it when it is too narrow.

**Position of the patient**

Supine, comfortable and relaxed.

**Position of the practitioner**

Seated at and facing the patient's head, on the side opposite the lesion.

**Points of contact**

On the cephalic hand, the thumb is placed on the orbital margin of the frontal bone and the index finger behind the frontozygomatic articulation. The other (inactive) fingers are spread out on the cranium.

The caudal hand controls the facial bones as follows:

— index finger on the superior border of the zygoma;

— middle finger on its inferior border;

— thumb on the orbital margin of the maxilla.

**Movement**

During the expansion phase, the cephalic hand enlarges the orbit in the following manner: the thumb draws the orbital margin of the frontal cephalad while the index finger pushes the frontozygomatic articulation anteriorly.

At the same time, the fingers of the caudal hand perform the following movements:

— index finger externally rotates the orbital border of the zygoma;

— middle finger accentuates this movement by pushing caudally and medially;

— thumb draws the orbital border of the maxilla caudally.

During the relaxation phase, these fingers gently resist the return to a neutral position.

These movements are repeated until a release is perceived.

**Comment**

This technique, which is easy to perform, nevertheless requires precise coordination of all the fingers.

Variation

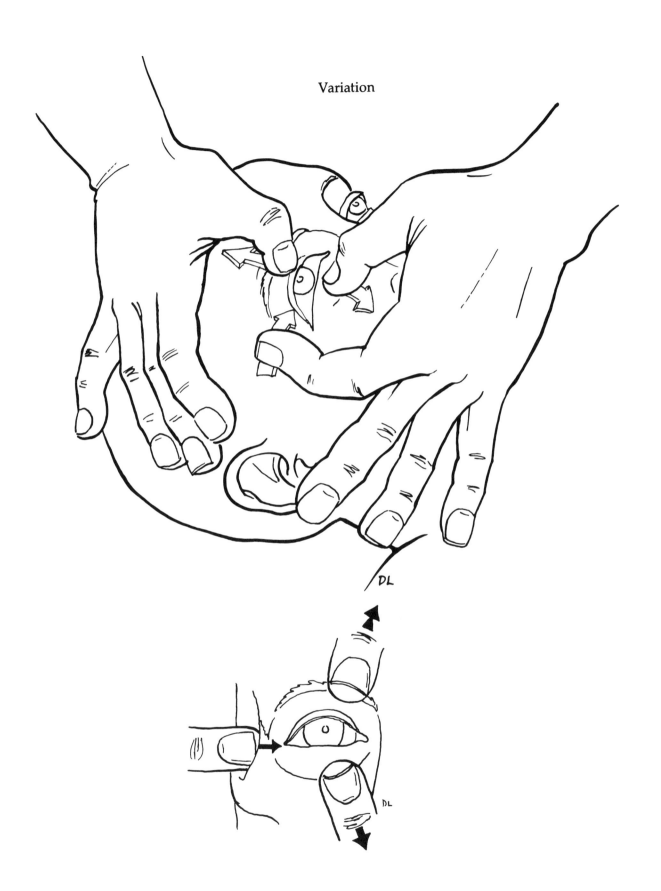

# REPOSITIONING OF THE LACRIMAL BONE

## Objective

To restore the functional relationship of the lacrimal bone between the external aspect of the ethmoid in the orbit and the frontal process of the maxilla, an important element in the drainage of the lacrimal canal.

## Position of the patient

Supine, comfortable and relaxed.

## Position of the practitioner

Seated beside the table, facing the patient at the patient's head.

## Points of contact

The cephalic hand controls the sphenoid. The clamp of the thumb and index finger cups the frontal while leaving it free; the terminal phalanges of thumb and index finger are positioned on the greater wings.

The pad of the thumb's terminal phalanx on the caudal hand is bent slightly and placed on the accessible part of the lacrimal bone.

## Movement

During the expansion phase, the cephalic hand draws the sphenoid in flexion (greater wings caudad and anterior), while the thumb of the caudal hand pushes the lacrimal anteriorly and very slightly laterally.

During the relaxation phase, the practitioner performs the reverse movement.

These movements are repeated until a release is perceived.

## Comment

The small external surface of the lacrimal requires that the practitioner make precise contact. The practitioner should particularly avoid pressing on the pulley of the superior oblique muscle of the eye, situated in front of and slightly above the eye itself.

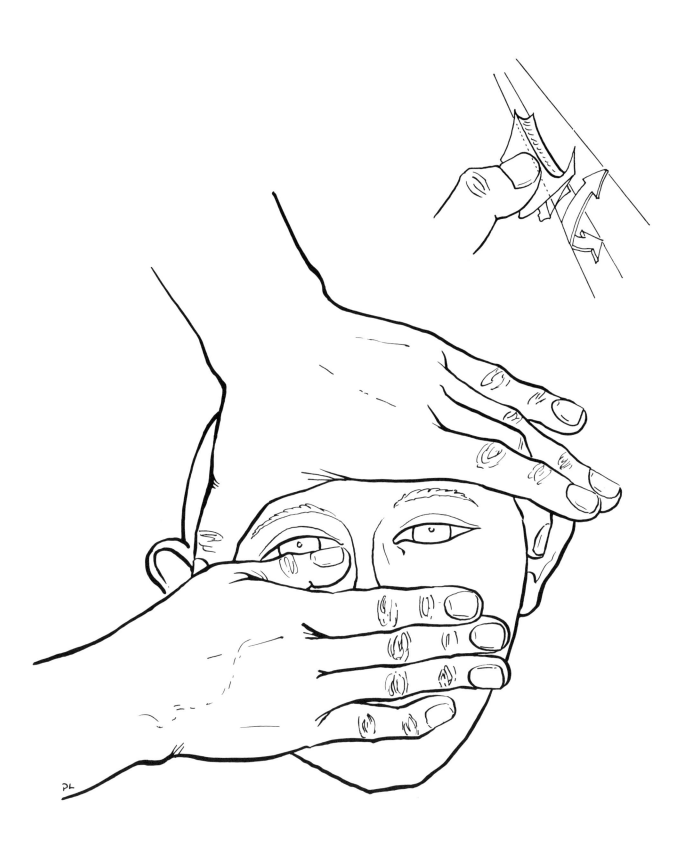

# VIII  Circulatory Techniques

Some techniques have a major circulatory effect. We have described a few of them in the preceding chapters of this book, such as the petrojugular technique (affecting systemic circulation) on page 92; the parietal lift (affecting arterial flow) on page 142; and the sphenopetrosal technique (affecting the cavernous sinuses) on page 108.

The following are some other, lesser known circulatory techniques which are nonetheless useful to the practitioner.

# COMPRESSION AT THE ASTERION

**Objective**

To perform an alternating compression and decompression that will have a profound effect on the circulation.

**Position of the patient**

Supine, comfortable and relaxed.

**Position of the practitioner**

Seated at the patient's head, forearms resting on the treatment table which has been adjusted to a convenient height.

**Points of contact**

The practitioner's hands are joined, fingers interlaced under the occiput. The practitioner's hands thus form a cradle to receive the occipital squama, with the thenar eminences placed on the asterions.

**Movement**

The practitioner, using the action of the deep flexor muscles of the fingers, exerts a gentle, progressive and continuous pressure during the expansion phase.

The pressure likewise progressively diminishes during the relaxation phase.

This alternating maneuver is applied over several cranial cycles until a release is perceived.

**Comment**

The execution of this technique is not difficult. The two compression points must, however, be carefully noted, since they are not necessarily symmetrical.

This maneuver involves the same combination of counter-indications as the compression of the fourth ventricle (page 46).

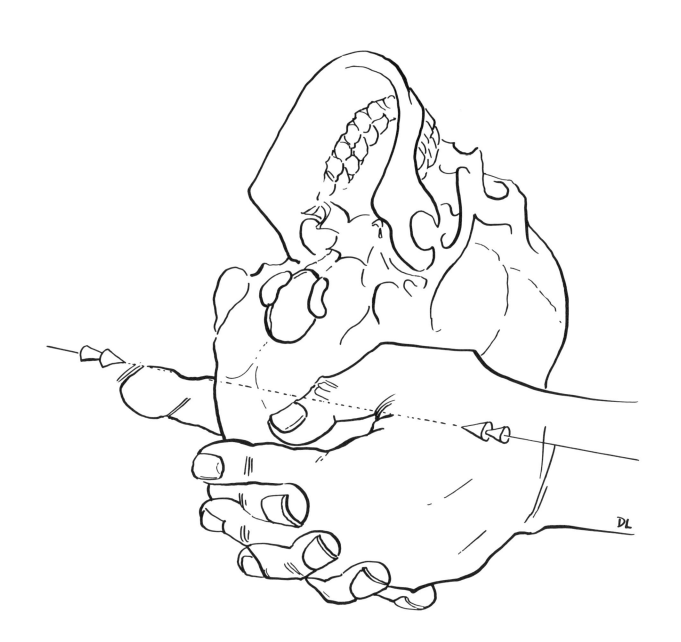

# IMMEDIATE GENERAL DECONGESTION

**Objective**

When well executed, this technique brings rapid, general relief of congestion throughout the cranium.

**Position of the patient**

Supine, comfortable and relaxed.

**Position of the practitioner**

Seated at the patient's head, forearms resting on the treatment table which has been adjusted to a convenient height.

**Points of contact**

On each side of the head, the practitioner places:
— the palm of the hand on the parietal bone, with the thenar and hypothenar eminences framing the parietal eminence;
— the index finger along the anterior border of the mastoid process, with the middle finger behind the latter;
— the little finger on the occipital squama;
— the thumb on the frontal bone.

**Movement**

During the expansion phase, the practitioner asks the patient to inhale slowly and deeply while drawing him or herself upwards, toward the practitioner. At the same time, the practitioner draws the mastoid process posteriorly and medially with the index fingers, and draws the occiput in flexion with the little fingers.

During the relaxation phase, the patient slowly exhales while tucking the head into the shoulder. At the same time, the practitioner pushes the mastoid process anteriorly and laterally with the index finger, and draws the occiput in extension with the little finger.

This maneuver is repeated until the feeling of congestion eases.

**Comment**

The success of this technique depends completely upon the cooperation of the patient.

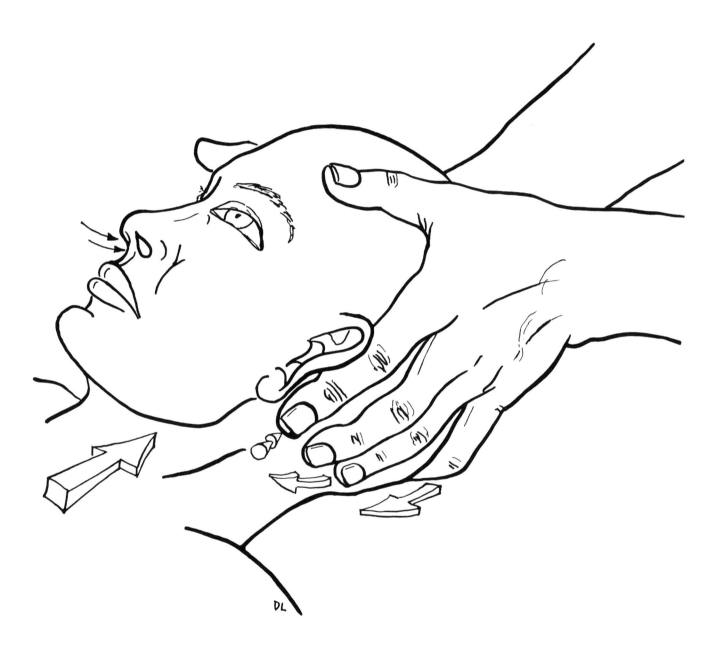

# RELEASE OF THE VASCULAR CANALS

**Objective**

To eliminate membranous tensions, thereby freeing the intracranial vascular canals.

**Position of the patient**

Supine, comfortable and relaxed.

**Position of the practitioner**

Seated at the patient's head, forearms resting on the treatment table which has been adjusted to a convenient height.

**Points of contact**

The technique described here is for the clinical situation in which the greater wing of the sphenoid is prominent and low on the right. If the greater wing is more prominent on the left, the hand positions are reversed.

The practitioner's hands are placed asymmetrically on the cranium. On the right hand, the thumb is placed along the mastoid process, with the thenar eminence on the mastoid portion. The other fingers are spread out on the occiput.

On the left hand, the thumb touches the left external surface of the greater wing of the sphenoid.

**Movement**

During the expansion phase:
—the right thumb gradually draws the mastoid process posteriorly and medially;
—at the same time, the left thumb moves the left greater wing of the sphenoid cephalad, posteriorly and medially.

When the relaxation phase begins, the practitioner's fingers (without releasing their contacts) permit a natural return to the neutral position.

These movements are repeated until a release is perceived.

**Comment**

While this technique can be used when neither great wing is markedly prominent, it is best to choose a side which appears more prominent.

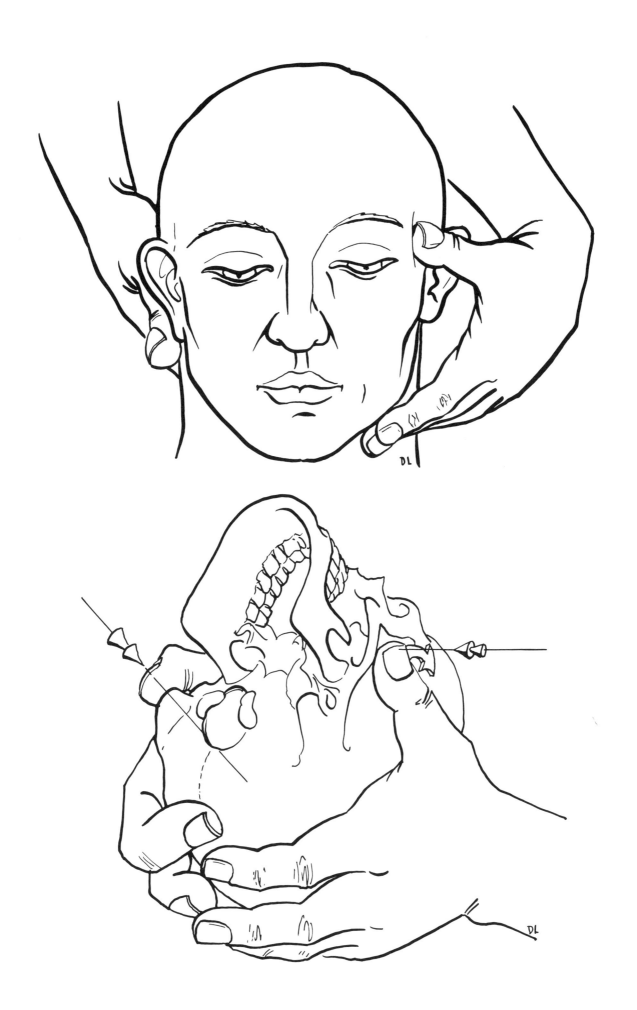

# GENERAL VASCULAR DRAINAGE

**Objective**

To relieve raised intracranial vascular pressure. This technique permits a more active drainage action than does the parietal lift (page 142).

**Position of the patient**

Supine, comfortable and relaxed.

**Position of the practitioner**

Seated either to the right or the left of the patient's head, the treatment table adjusted to a convenient height.

**Points of contact**

The intraoral index finger of the caudal hand contacts the palatine vault at the intermaxillary articulation.

The palm of the other hand cups the cranium as follows:

—thenar and hypothenar eminences on each side of the sagittal suture, on the parietals, behind the bregma;

—fingers spread out as widely as possible onto the occipital squama.

**Movement**

During the expansion phase:

—the intraoral index finger, its pad pressing toward the nostrils, carries along a movement of flexion;

—the thenar and hypothenar eminences depress the sagittal suture and move the antero-superior angles of the parietals posteriorly while the fingers push the occipital squama caudally.

During the relaxation phase, without releasing these contacts, the practitioner allows the cranial mechanism to return to a neutral position.

This rhythmic maneuver must be repeated until a release is perceived.

**Comment**

The discriminating action of each finger of the cephalic hand in following subtle variations in the motion is the key to the success of this technique.

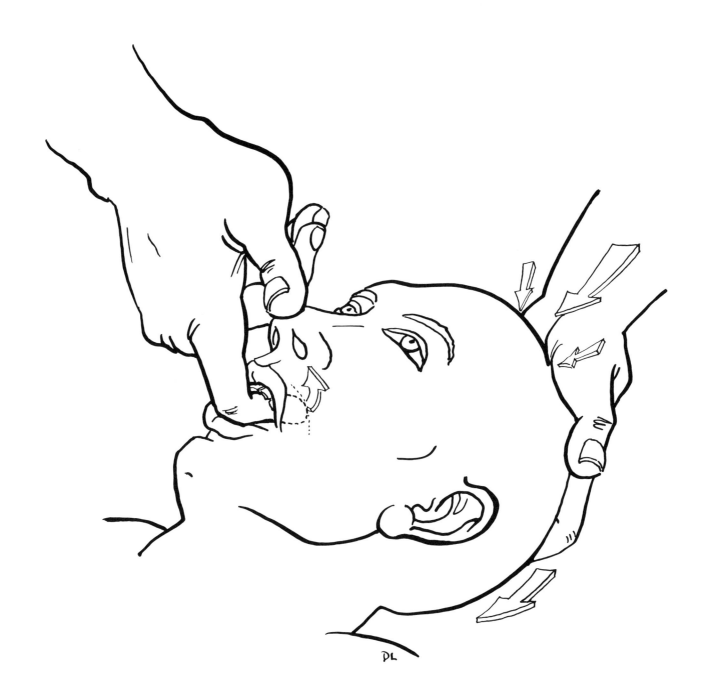

# GENERAL VASCULAR DRAINAGE

## FRONTOPARIETO-OCCIPITAL APPROACH

**Objective**

To relieve raised intracranial vascular pressure. This technique is applied when medical reasons prohibit exerting the pressure of the intrabuccal index finger on the palate.

**Position of the patient**

Supine, comfortable and relaxed.

**Position of the practitioner**

Seated either to the right or the left of the patient's head, the treatment table adjusted to a convenient height.

**Points of contact**

The anterior caudal hand is placed on the forehead as follows:
— palm covering the metopic suture;
— fingers passing over the coronal suture to open out on the anterior portion of the parietals.

The cephalic hand touches the posterior part of the cranium:
— heel on the posterior portion of the parietals, with thenar and hypothenar eminences on either side of the sagittal suture;
— fingers on the occipital squama.

**Movement**

During the expansion phase:
— the palm of the caudal hand draws the frontal cephalad and posteriorly in the direction of the vertex, the fingers accentuating the anterior depression of the parietals;
— with the heel of the other hand, the practitioner performs the same maneuver on the posterior portion of the parietals, the fingers increasing the flexion of the occipital squama.

During the relaxation phase, without releasing these contacts, the practitioner allows the cranial mechanism to return to a neutral position.

This rhythmic maneuver is repeated until a release is perceived.

**Comment**

The inexperienced practitioner may encounter some difficulty in performing this technique, especially in executing the precise movements of the fingers.

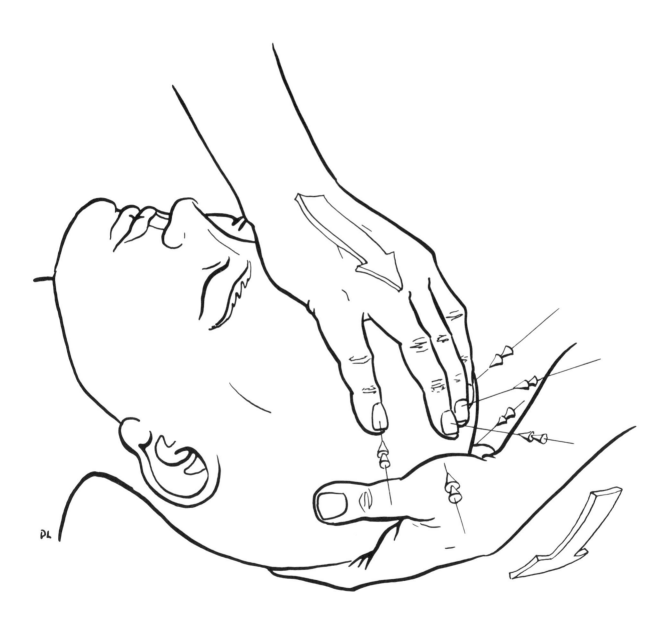

# GENERAL VASCULAR DRAINAGE
## FRONTO-OCCIPITAL APPROACH

### Objectives

- To amplify the general motion of the cranium and thereby improve its internal circulation.
- To induce a pumping action at the articulation of petrous and basiocciput so as to increase the cranial drainage via the internal jugular vein.

### Position of the patient

Supine, comfortable and relaxed.

### Position of the practitioner

Seated either to the right or the left of the patient's head, the table adjusted to a convenient height.

### Points of contact

The caudal hand, positioned transversely, cups the occipital squama. The thumb and index finger are placed on the anterior border of the mastoid processes.

The palm of the cephalic hand envelops the frontal. The thumb and index and/or middle fingers make contact on the greater wings of the sphenoid.

### Movement

During the expansion phase:
— the patient inhales slowly and deeply while stretching out the axial skeleton as much as possible;
— the thumb and index finger of the practitioner's caudal hand draw the mastoid process posteriorly and medially;
— at the same time, the cephalic hand accentuates the flexion movements of the frontal and the sphenoid.

During the relaxation phase:
— the patient exhales slowly while tucking the head into the shoulders;
— the practitioner draws the mastoid processes anteriorly and laterally with the caudal hand, while assisting the extension movement of the frontal and the sphenoid with the cephalic hand.

These movements are repeated until a release is perceived.

In an acceptable variation, the practitioner may assume a passive role during the relaxation phase, but must take care not to release any points of contact.

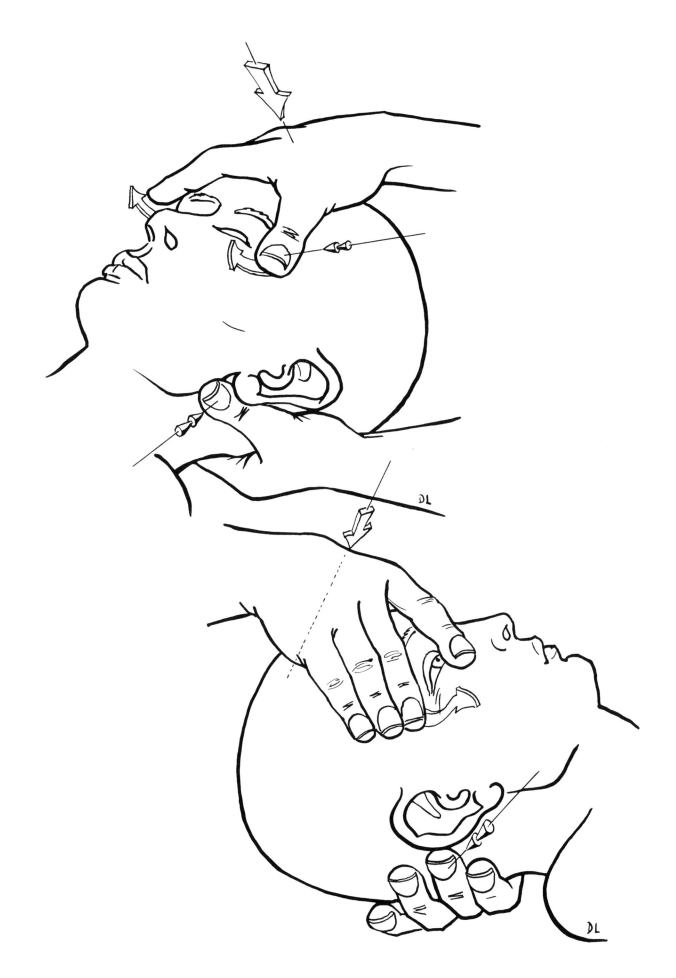

# DRAINAGE OF THE POSTERIOR FOSSA

**Objective**

To activate the drainage of the posterior fossa of the cranium and, in particular, that of the lateral sinuses.

**Position of the patient**

Supine, comfortable and relaxed.

**Position of the practitioner**

Seated at the patient's head, forearms resting on the treatment table which has been adjusted to a convenient height.

**Points of contact**

The practitioner's hands are joined under the occiput, fingers interlaced, forming a cradle to receive the occipital squama. The thenar eminences are placed at the posteroinferior angles of the parietals (at the asterion). The thumbs lie along the mastoid processes.

**Movement**

During the expansion phase, simultaneously:
— the thenar eminences gradually compress the posteroinferior angles of the parietals;
— the thumbs draw the mastoid processes posteriorly and medially.

During the relaxation phase, the practitioner (without releasing any contacts) allows the cranial mechanism to return to a neutral position.

This maneuver must cease as soon as the patient feels a sensation of warmth in the posterior part of the cranium.

**Comment**

Generally, this technique is to be applied before more specific techniques, such as those that treat petrojugular and sphenopetrosal problems.

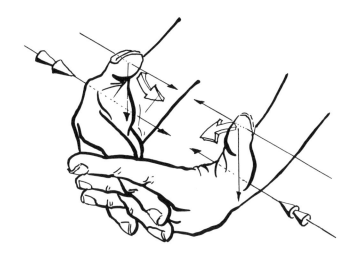

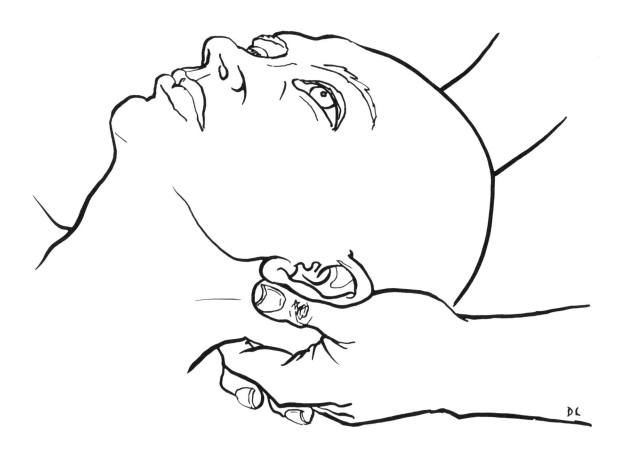

# DRAINAGE OF THE SAGITTAL SINUS

**Objective**

To increase the physiological activity of the sagittal sinus when it is restricted or reduced.

**Position of the patient**

Supine, comfortable and relaxed.

**Position of the practitioner**

Seated at the patient's head, forearms resting on the treatment table which has been adjusted to a convenient height.

**Points of contact**

The practitioner uses a somewhat modified vault hold.

Both thumbs are crossed above the sagittal suture and make their points of contact on the posterosuperior angles of the opposite parietals. The other fingers are positioned on both sides of the ear, along the inferior border of each parietal.

**Movement**

During the expansion phase, the practitioner lifts the parietals (see the earlier description of this technique on page 142) with the last four fingers of both hands. At the same time, the practitioner presses his or her thumbs on the posterosuperior angles laterally and synchronously until a release is perceived under the thumbs.

During the relaxation phase, the practitioner's fingers are passive.

The practitioner repeats this technique as necessary, moving the thumbs to restricted areas along the sagittal suture from the back to the front.

**Comment**

The practitioner must perfectly coordinate the action of the thumbs with that of the other fingers. Moreover, the two phases of this technique must be synchronized with those of the cranial mechanism.

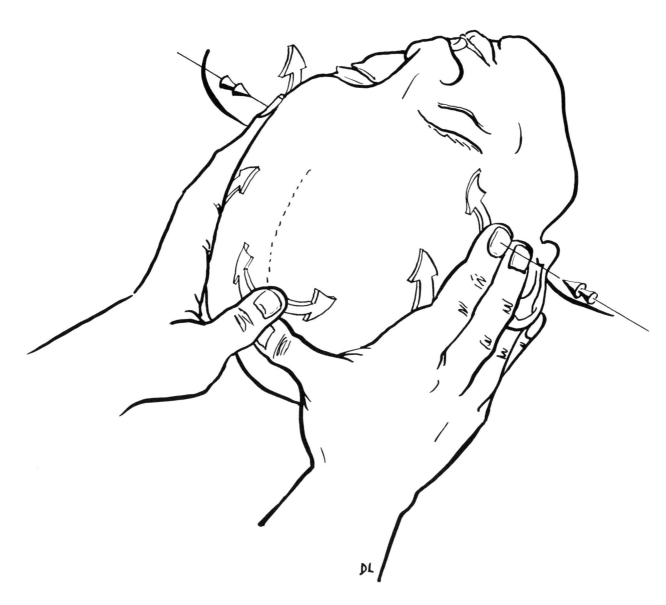

# DRAINAGE OF THE PTERYGOID PLEXI

## Objective

To increase the physiological activity of the pterygoid venous plexi, which play an essential part in the drainage of the face.

## Position of the patient

Supine, comfortable and relaxed, head turned to the side opposite the lesion.

## Position of the practitioner

Seated at the patient's head, on the side of the lesion, the table adjusted to a convenient height.

## Points of contact

The cephalic hand immobilizes the head as follows:
— palm of the hand against the parietal;
— thumb and index finger on the temporal surrounding the ear;
— other fingers spread out on the frontal.
The caudal hand envelops the patient's mandible, holding it in the palm.

## Movement

The practitioner initiates a series of slow, rhythmic movements with the caudal hand. The movements increase the discharge from the pterygoid sinuses.

## Comment

As with any circulatory maneuver, the practitioner must:
— precede it with an "up-stream" preparatory technique (petrojugular, sphenopetrosal, etc.);
— continue the action long enough to make it effective.

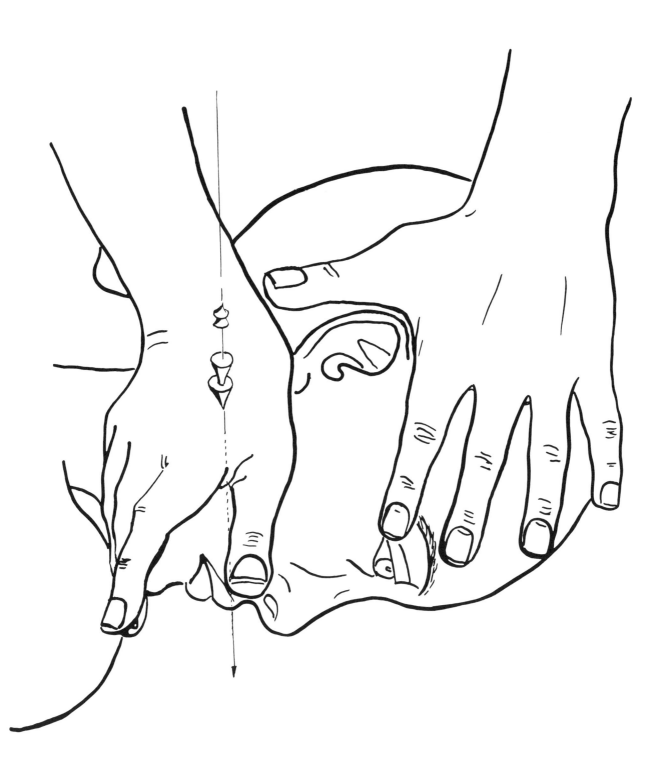